Aromatherapy *and*

HERBAL REMEDIES

FOR PREGNANCY, BIRTH, AND BREASTFEEDING

Demetria Clark

Healthy Living Publications
SUMMERTOWN, TENNESSEE

Library of Congress Cataloging-in-Publication Data

Clark, Demetria.
  Aromatherapy and herbal remedies for pregnancy, birth, and breastfeeding /
Demetria Clark.
    pages cm
  Includes index.
  ISBN 978-1-57067-328-3 (pbk.) — ISBN 978-1-57067-866-0 (e-book)
1. Pregnancy.   2. Herbs--Therapeutic use.   3. Pregnancy—Nutritional
aspects.   I. Title.
  RG525.C643 2015
  615.82068—dc23

                                                            2015024048

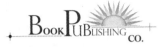

Book Publishing Company is a member of Green Press Initiative. We chose to
print this title on FSC-certified paper with 100 percent postconsumer recycled
content, processed without chlorine, which saves the following natural resources:

43 trees

1,340 pounds of solid waste

20,020 gallons of water

3,691 pounds of greenhouse gases

19 million BTUs of energy

For more information on Green Press Initiative, visit greenpressinitiative.org.

Environmental impact estimates were made using the Environmental Defense
Fund Paper Calculator. For more information, visit papercalculator.org.

Printed on recycled paper

Cover and interior design: John Wincek
Stock photography: 123 RF

Printed in Canada

Book Publishing Company
PO Box 99
Summertown, TN 38483
888-260-8458
bookpubco.com

ISBN: 978-1-57067-328-3

The information in this book is
presented for educational purposes only. It isn't intended to
be a substitute for the medical
advice of a physician or other
health care professional.

20 19 18 17 16 15   1 2 3 4 5 6 7 8 9

Contents

Acknowledgments   iv
Introduction   v

Chapter 1
Introduction to Aromatherapy and Essential Oils   1

Chapter 2
Essential Oils for Pregnancy, Labor, and Breastfeeding   17

Chapter 3
Introduction to Herbal Remedies   29

Chapter 4
Herbs for Pregnancy, Labor, and Breastfeeding   49

Chapter 5
Making Your Own Aromatherapy and Herbal Remedies   77

Chapter 6
Remedies for Pregnancy   89

Chapter 7
Remedies for Labor and Delivery   133

Chapter 8
Remedies for Breastfeeding and Other Postpartum Concerns   145

Glossary   171
Suppliers   173
Associations and Schools   175
Recommended Reading   176
Index   177

Acknowledgments

I must thank my family, my husband, and my children.
You are the first in my heart, my life, and my being.
My gratefulness knows no bounds;
I appreciate you, love you, and am blessed to have you.
I am also blessed to have a large, funny, supportive,
and close extended family;
I am so thankful for your support and love.
I also greatly appreciate all the women I have worked with
over the years; each has educated me in some way,
shared with me, and taught me more than I can express.
Thank you for your trust and support.

Introduction

n this book I share the remedies I've used and the insights I've gained from my experience with birth. My extensive herbal and aromatherapy knowledge offers alternative solutions for the issues you may be having related to pregnancy, birth, and the very early days of motherhood. I ask only that if you use any of these remedies, you advise your midwife or doctor.

I am first and foremost a mother and a wife. Because my own family is the center of my world, I have felt privileged to work as a doula (birth coach) and then midwife for over twelve years. I also have been a practicing aromatherapist and herbalist for more than twenty years. I believe in relying on natural methods first; this is something that I have believed in since childhood. As a child, I moved with my family all over the United States, and I had the chance to hear old-time stories about healing and see how other cultures and families handled health issues. My own mother believed that healthy foods, fresh air, and sunshine led to healthy children.

I was raised to see birth and pregnancy as normal and natural. A pivotal moment for me was attending a home birth when I was fifteen years old. It was so beautiful and left such an impression on me, I knew I would be assisting mothers in my future.

The oldest of five children, I am eighteen years older than my youngest sibling. In my family, all the women gave birth naturally—to many children. Because they had pretty smooth pregnancies and labors, it never occurred to me that my pregnancies could go another way. And I was right. I always joke that I was too naive to not trust my body; I never considered not following my instincts. Today, with children who are almost adults, I still follow my instincts.

Although I follow my gut, I am by nature a very solution-based and practical woman. My confidence as an herbalist comes from the knowledge that many herbs have had hundreds, if not thousands, of years of recorded use. Many systems of herbalism have well-documented materia medicas, including traditional Chinese medicine and Ayurveda.

The trend today is to ask if scientific studies can validate traditional practices. The fact is, most herbs and essential oils have not been adequately studied by modern methods. In my experience, many studies are unreliable anyway, and recommendations are likely to change as a result of the next study. So I believe in being practical. If a woman can safely eat an herb during pregnancy, it is probably safe overall, potentially less so in high dosages. Consider basil, for example. Many sources say that it is not safe in high doses. Yet I know that one cup or more of basil may go into one serving of pesto, and it's safe for a pregnant woman to eat pesto. Therefore, I use basil in herbal remedies designed to be used during pregnancy. Again, on a practical note, I tell clients that if any remedy (or food, for that matter) makes them feel funny or ill, they should stop using it.

Based on my extensive experience, I have several other bits of advice for expecting or new mothers:

ALWAYS EVALUATE WHETHER SOMETHING IS BENEFICIAL TO YOU. Ask the following questions: Is what I am consuming or using beneficial to my baby? Is that essential oil or herb safe for pregnancy? The listings of essential oils in chapters 2 and herbs in chapter 4 will help you answer these questions.

MAKE INFORMED CHOICES. Yes, you have choices about how to manage your pregnancy and your baby's birth. For example, will you rely on a midwife or a physician? Be willing to do the research that is necessary for you to feel comfortable with your choices.

CHOOSE YOUR CAREGIVER CAREFULLY. Except in emergency situations, you choose who you want to provide your care. If you do not feel you and your care provider work well together, understand each other, and have a good honest relationship, then find another care provider. Find someone you work well with and who supports your birth plan and priorities. Educate yourself about the practices and ideals of any care provider. For example, would you choose a physician who has a 60 percent C-section rate?

INTERVIEW PROSPECTIVE CAREGIVERS. If you seek an aromatherapist, herbalist, massage therapist, or other care provider, find a few to call and interview them about their practice style, rates, education, and previous experience with pregnant clients. Ask if they have specialized training dealing with pregnancy issues. Practitioners should not be rude when you question them about their skill sets. Most love to talk about their education, experiences, and the traditions they follow. Just keep in mind that herbal and aromatherapy education in the United States is not standardized. I have met many fine herbalists and aromatherapists who studied for years and are completely self-taught.

BE HONEST WITH YOUR CAREGIVER. Always tell your midwife or doctor about any remedies you are using. This includes aromatherapy, herbs, prescription drugs, supplements, and over-the-counter products, including those that are applied topically. This is important because some substances are not safe to use together. Others may have undesirable side effects. By sharing this information, you can avoid potential problems for you and your baby.

TRUST YOURSELF. This is your baby and your body. You are the expert about how you feel. Listen to your own needs. By doing so, you are ensuring a safer pregnancy.

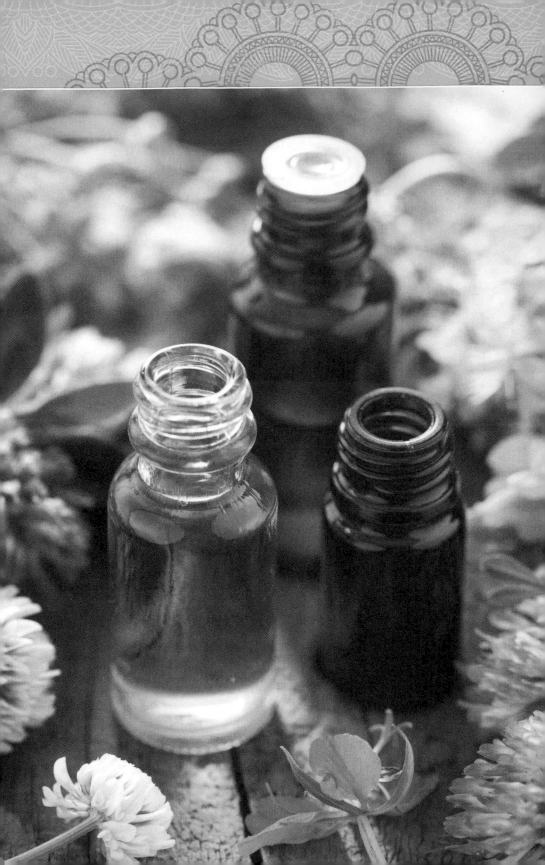

Introduction to Aromatherapy and Essential Oils

Aromatherapy, simply defined, is the process of using scents for healing. It's a very easy and practical everyday therapy to use at home; in fact, many types of aromatherapy applications can be made at home (see chapter 5, "Making Your Own Aromatherapy and Herbal Remedies," pages 77 to 87). Topical applications, which are applied directly to the skin, include body sprays, compresses, creams, liniments, and massage oils. Alternatively, scents can be diffused into the surrounding air or dispersed through steam and inhaled.

Essential oils are the keystones of aromatherapy. Using essential oils singly or in combination can bring both healing and comfort anytime; during pregnancy, labor, and the postpartum period, these plant-based oils can be particularly gentle, safe, and effective.

Aromatherapy remedies can be used cosmetically as well as to target deeper issues, such as specific physical, emotional, and mental health concerns. Aromatherapy works because the system involved in the sense of smell, the olfactory system, connects the nose with points in the brain that comprise the limbic system. Here lies the amygdala, hippocampus, and hypothalamus, parts of the brain that are concerned primarily with emotion and motivation. When stimulated by smell, the limbic system releases chemicals that affect the central nervous system, influencing physical, emotional, and mental health.

The term "aromatherapy" was coined in 1928 by chemist René-Maurice Gattefossé, who was inspired to study and write about essential oils after an explosion in his lab. His hand was badly burned, and he treated his wounds with lavender essential oil. When his burns healed remarkably quickly, he decided to investigate essential oils further.

Influenced by the work of Gattefossé, French physician Jean Valnet used essential oils as antiseptics while treating wounded soldiers during World War II. He continued his use and scientific study of essential oils, eventually publishing his classic text, *L'armathérapy*, in France in 1964. The English version, *The Practice of Aromatherapy*, is still available. Valnet's approach of matching the healing properties of a specific plant with the needs of the patient remains the backbone of modern aromatherapy. His work has inspired many well-known aromatherapists, including Micheline Arcier, Julia Lawless, Marguerite Mary, Shirley Price, Robert Tisserand, and me.

From our own individual experiences, we know that anything we smell in our natural environment can stimulate sometimes strong reactions. The powerful sense of smell can evoke attachments, feelings, and memories. For example, scent attracts people to potential mates and promotes a bond between a new baby and its parents. In fact, whether we're aware of it or not, the sense of smell activates our most primal emotions, including fear, love, and lust.

Each brain processes scent differently. For example, the scent of lavender typically makes people feel relaxed and at ease. However, for some people, lavender may smell unpleasant, or it may cause them to feel agitated or restless. It's important that anyone who uses aromatherapy, whether a professional aromatherapist or someone who occasionally uses a diffuser at home, be aware that scents don't elicit the same reactions in every aromatherapy user. When using aromatherapy during pregnancy, it's essential to remember that the sense of smell can be much more acute during this time.

ESSENTIAL OILS

Essential oils are concentrated plant oils. Despite the name, essential oils are not all that oily because they're not true oils but rather the essence of plant components. Essential oils are found in the flowers, fruits, leaves, roots, seeds, and stems of plants. Most are clear, but some are amber, brown, orange, or yellow, depending on the color of the plant source.

There are different ways to extract an essential oil from a plant. The most common method is distillation. Other essential oils are expressed, and some are extracted using ancient techniques. Following are some common extraction methods:

DISTILLATION. The most popular method of obtaining essential oils is through steam distillation. Anyone who is familiar with how an old-fashioned moonshine still works knows the basics of distillation: water is heated to the boiling point, then the resulting steam passes through fresh plant material that has been placed above the boiling water. The steam pressure is carefully controlled. When the steam passes through the plant material, it causes the plant's cell walls to swell and break down. This allows the essential oil to be released as vapor. Then the essential oil vapor and water pass through a condenser that cools the steam and the oil into a liquid. Because essential oils don't dissolve in water, the two can be separated. Essential oils that are lighter than water rise to the top and are then siphoned off. Essential oils that are heavier than water sink to the bottom and can be collected.

ENFLEURAGE. An ancient technique for extracting essential oils is enfleurage, which involves the application of odorless fats and oils to plants to absorb the plants' essential scent qualities. In the past, this process was typically used to extract the essential oils of highly scented, fatty flowers, such as honeysuckle and jasmine. This method is not commonly used in the making of modern essential oils.

EXPRESSION. Expression is a method that physically forces the essential oil from a plant. For example, components of a citrus plant may be pressed to obtain the essential oil. You can witness an example of expression simply by peeling an orange. When you bend the rind, the orange's essential oil sprays forth, creating a visible display (if you look closely) and coating your fingers with an enticing scent. Expression is also known as cold-pressing, and the resulting oils may be referred to as cold-pressed extractions.

ABSOLUTES AND HYDROSOLS

Essential oils aren't the only plant products used in aromatherapy. Two other ingredients used in aromatherapy are absolutes and hydrosols:

ABSOLUTE. Despite the fact that absolutes are often displayed and sold right beside essential oils, an absolute is not considered a pure essential oil but instead falls into a classification of its own. An absolute is obtained through chemical solvent extraction. The solvent used is alcohol, and the alcohol is removed with vacuum extraction. The most common absolutes are jasmine, rose, and sandalwood. Jasmine absolute is one of my favorites to use during the postpartum period.

HYDROSOL. When an essential oil is produced by distillation, the aromatic water that remains is the hydrosol. While essential oils should be diluted for topical use, hydrosols are more dilute and considered safe for topical use without dilution. Hydrosols are commonly sold wherever essential oils are sold and can be safely added to all kinds of hair- and skin-care products, such as creams, facial toners, liniments, and lotions.

AROMATHERAPY APPLICATIONS

Essential oils can be used in bath salts, body sprays, liniments, massage oils, salves, and many more wonderful topical applications. They also can be healing when diffused into the air or inhaled. To learn how to make essential oil therapies at home, see the basic methods in chapter 5 (pages 77 to 87) and the remedies in chapters 6, 7, and 8 (pages 89 to 169).

Note that some essential oils should not be used during pregnancy (see page 22). Others should not be used in general (see page 23). It's critical to always check when it's safe to use a specific essential oil, because one may be safe during the postpartum period but not during pregnancy, for example.

APPLYING ESSENTIAL OILS TOPICALLY

Because they can be very strong, with few exceptions, essential oils should be diluted before being applied to the skin. Dilution is the best way to prevent reactions or sensitivities. Typically, essential oils are diluted with a carrier oil, such as a nut, seed, or vegetable oil (see box, page 14). When it's safe to apply an essential oil directly to the skin, it is said that the oil can be applied "neat," or without dilution.

Body Sprays

Body sprays are used to tone the skin, and they can be quite cooling and refreshing. In addition, their effects can go much deeper. They can effectively lift moods, energize, and ease anxiety or stress. Body sprays are very easy to make and use.

Compresses

A compress is made by soaking a piece of clean cloth (such as linen, cotton, or gauze) or a washcloth in hot or cold water mixed with one or more essential oils. Extraordinarily easy to make and immediately soothing, compresses have a multitude of uses for the expecting or new mother. They can be used to treat hemorrhoids, varicose veins, muscle pain, sore breasts, and tissues that can be torn or bruised during birth.

Creams and Lotions

Any cream or lotion that you already have can be enhanced with essential oils. Ideally, mix essential oils with an unscented cream or lotion, using a brand that works well for you. Most people prefer to apply a light cream on the body and a thick cream on the face (especially overnight) or on dry skin anywhere on the body. Because skin stretches and can be sensitive during pregnancy, healing creams can bring needed relief.

Liniments

A liniment is a combination of an essential oil and food-grade alcohol, such as vodka, or witch hazel. Liniments are rubbed into the skin to provide relief from sore muscles, strains, and inflammations of the ligaments, muscles, and tendons. An expecting mother, for example, would welcome a liniment to control her back pain as her body grows and changes.

Massage Oils

Massage oils are made by combining a carrier oil (see box, page 14) and essential oils or infused oils. A gentle massage done with a beautifully scented massage oil can do wonders by promoting relaxation and calm.

Salves

A salve has a firmer texture than a cream or lotion and is made by combining essential oils and beeswax, coconut oil, or another firm base. Like creams and lotions, salves are applied directly to the skin to treat physical ailments. They can also be helpful in treating emotional issues. For example, one salve can prevent stretch marks and another can promote a restful sleep.

INHALING ESSENTIAL OILS

Perhaps one of the simplest forms of aromatherapy is inhalation. This involves breathing in, or inhaling, an essential oil to obtain the oil's healing benefits. The essential oil travels through the nose and mouth to the lungs, making inhalation an especially great form of therapy for head colds and sinus ailments. Simply removing the bottle cap and inhaling an essential oil can be therapeutic, particularly to aid breathing.

One of the simplest and most effective ways to receive the benefit of essential oils is to smell them. Open the cap and take a sniff. Or put a few drops on a handkerchief that you can carry with you. You can use essential oils this way anytime, anywhere. Here are two other easy applications that will allow you to enjoy essential oils with almost no effort:

- Make a natural air freshener spray to use at home, at work, or in the car. Put 2 ounces of pure water in a mist spray bottle and add 50 to 75 drops of an essential oil. Put the spray cap on the bottle. Shake well before spraying into the air. I use this application in the car and in the living room, places that tend to get a little stinky thanks to my two sons.

- Add 25 drops of one or more essential oils to a bowl of potpourri that has lost its scent. Or create your own potpourri by adding drops of an essential oil to dried leaves, flowers, and so on. Mix together in a container, cover tightly, and store for several days to allow the potpourri to absorb the essential oil.

When you want a portable remedy, add a few drops of essential oil to a small bottle that contains a few large grains of rock salt. For example, use peppermint essential oil to avoid dizziness and fainting, which can be a concern during pregnancy. If you anticipate stressful events, use clary sage, grapefruit, lavender, mandarin, or sweet orange essential oils to keep calm.

For anyone who has a cold or allergies, a quick remedy to relieve congestion or enhance respiratory function is to inhale essential oils in steam. For example, the over-the-bowl method involves boiling water, pouring it into a bowl, and adding 3 to 7 drops of essential oil. Lean over the bowl, place a towel over your head and the bowl (forming a makeshift tent to contain the steam), and inhale for about 5 minutes. To avoid burns, be careful not to get your face too close to the water or the steam and avoid knocking over the bowl.

DIFFUSING ESSENTIAL OILS

When an essential oil is diffused, it's dispersed into the surrounding air with a device called a diffuser. Diffusing is considered one of the most effective ways to deliver the healing benefits of essential oils in aromatherapy. Many positive effects can be obtained through diffusion (see box, opposite page).

Note that a humidifier is *not* an essential oil diffuser, although many people use essential oils in humidifiers at the risk of damaging

BENEFITS OF USING ESSENTIAL OILS IN A DIFFUSER

Diffusing essential oils creates the following effects:

- Cleans and purifies the air, discouraging the growth of bacteria, mold, viruses, and other pathogens
- Boosts the immune system and overall wellness
- Helps to increase concentration and focus
- Promotes feelings of peace and well-being by increasing the negative ions in the atmosphere
- Positively affects mood and emotional health
- Lessens anxiety and stress
- Bonus! Makes your house smell wonderful

either its plastic or electronic parts. Rather, an essential oil diffuser is a device designed specifically to break down the oil particles and disperse them in the air. Using a diffuser is ideal but not necessary; simply putting an essential oil on a cotton ball or in a sachet will allow the scent and benefits to spread over time.

When using an essential oil diffuser, be sure to use only pure essential oils. If you use anything artificial, you will be at risk of breathing in chemicals and synthetics. Feel free to try different diffusers; you may find that you prefer a certain type for a specific application. Mix it up. Many varieties of diffusers are available; be sure to adhere to the diffuser manufacturer's instructions for adding essential oils. Following are descriptions of various types of diffusers:

CANDLE DIFFUSER. I did an informal poll of more than two thousand people, including my students and readers of my books, and the candle diffuser seems to be the most popular kind of diffuser. An inexpensive form of heat diffuser, a candle diffuser typically uses a tea-light candle to heat a small bowl made of a substance that is safe to use with essential oils, such as ceramic, glass, or soapstone. The small candle heats the bowl and voilà—scent is released into the air.

EVAPORATIVE DIFFUSER. As the name indicates, this type of diffuser employs the use of evaporation. A fan in the diffuser blows air through a pad or filter that has a few drops of essential oil on it. The air blowing through the pad causes the essential oil to evaporate.

HEAT DIFFUSER. Like an evaporative diffuser, a heat diffuser uses evaporation as the dispersal method; however, heat is faster than evaporation when it comes to diffusing essential oils. A heat diffuser may use a candle or light bulb to warm an essential oil and release its scent.

NEBULIZING DIFFUSER. Unlike an ultrasonic diffuser, a nebulizing diffuser doesn't need the addition of water but instead diffuses pure essential oil directly into the air by breaking it up into super-tiny molecules. This type of diffuser is considered superior because it releases the entire oil into the air in very fine particles. In fact, a nebulizing diffuser is thought to be the most effective and therapeutic kind of diffuser available.

ULTRASONIC DIFFUSER. Typically requiring the addition of water, an ultrasonic diffuser generates a fine mist and sends tiny oil particles into the air. A few drops of essential oil are added to the water in the device, making the diffuser economical to run. Some even have timers. Because it adds moisture to the air, this method of diffusion can be particularly beneficial during the dry winter months or in dry climates.

ESSENTIAL OIL SAFETY

Essential oils, like any other substance that is used therapeutically, should be handled properly. Purchase them with care, use them with knowledge, and store them so they will last. Useful guidelines for buying, using, and storing essential oils follow.

BUYING ESSENTIAL OILS

Choosing an essential oil—or an essential oil company to purchase from—deserves careful consideration. My advice is to evaluate each essential oil individually; don't assume that if you like a certain essential oil company, you'll always prefer its oils. Although some people swear by one supplier, my essential oil cupboard is stocked with a variety of brands because I always take the time to research each individual essential oil I purchase. Fortunately, there is no shortage of reliable essential oil suppliers, and most will answer questions and welcome customer feedback.

Essential oils can be found in stores or online. The advantage of purchasing in a store, of course, is that you can smell and feel the essential oil before purchasing it. And there are other important considerations. Here are some tips on how to buy essential oils:

DO YOUR HOMEWORK. Before you buy it—and before you use it—read about the essential oil that interests you. Check a few sources to confirm it's the right choice to meet your needs.

In North America and all over the world, essential oils begin as a crop on a farm. The crop is harvested and transported to a distillation facility, where the essential oils are made. Some companies produce their product from seed to bottle, but many do not.

This final product is then sold in bulk quantities on the commodities market. Naturally, based on their ingredients and production factors, essential oils will vary in price and quality. Although some companies claim to offer "therapeutic grade" essential oils, this is just a marketing term. There is no legal or industry standard definition of what a therapeutic grade essential oil is. No official international distinctions, standards, or grades exist; and no North American distinctions exist, either. Therefore, it's important to shop discriminately.

READ THE LABEL. Make sure that what you're buying is an actual pure essential oil. The label should list only the common and botanical (or Latin) name of the essential oil; for example, sweet orange essential oil (*Citrus sinensis*) or bitter orange essential oil (*Citrus aurantium*). Sometimes an essential oil is bottled with a carrier oil; if so, the label should be marked accordingly. Keep this in mind when you intend to buy a blend or a diluted essential oil.

Be wary of labels that feature potentially confusing or misleading terms, such as "fragrance oil," "nature identical oil," "perfume oil," or "therapeutic oil." When such terms appear on labels, they signal that the bottle contents are not pure, single essential oils. In addition, be leery of terms such as "aromatherapy grade," "medical grade," and "therapeutic grade." There are no formal standards or "grades" used in the industry, so the inclusion of such terms on a label may be intentionally misleading.

FOLLOW YOUR NOSE. If you're purchasing an essential oil at a store, smell the oil sample and make sure you like it. If the scent turns you off, listen to your senses and find an alternative. The good news is that in almost all cases you can find a different essential oil to meet your needs. You can always revisit the essential oil you didn't like at a later date.

Your ability to identify a high-quality oil will develop over time, as you gain experience. Look for (or sniff for) an essential oil that smells like the plant it's distilled from. If you can detect anything else, such as chemicals or fillers, pass on purchasing that particular essential oil.

FEEL THE ESSENTIAL OIL. When you're at a store looking at a sample, put a drop of essential oil on your finger and rub the oil between your finger and thumb. It should feel clean and not too oily. Some of the thicker, darker oils, such as patchouli and vetiver, can be more oily than lighter oils, such as lavender and sweet orange.

PICK PROPER PACKAGING. Choose essential oils that are packaged in dark bottles. Amber is the darkest, and that's what I prefer, although you can also find cobalt blue, green, and violet bottles, which are acceptable. Make sure the bottles are topped with orifice reducers and caps—not droppers, which erode over time and allow air to enter the bottles. Always avoid essential oils sold in plastic or clear glass bottles.

SHOP AROUND. Essential oils aren't inexpensive. Look around online and in stores to get a feel for reasonable costs. If you see a price that seems too good to be true, it probably is. When purchasing online, make sure all the essential oils aren't priced the same. Uniform pricing is a red flag that the seller may not be reputable, because different varieties of essential oils simply should not cost the same (see box, page 9).

USING ESSENTIAL OILS SAFELY

When it comes to essential oil safety, I always advise erring on the side of caution. While this book is a guide to using aromatherapy during pregnancy, labor, and the postpartum period, keep in mind that the general information provided in chapters 1, 2, and 5 give you the tools to use aromatherapy at home during other times and for other reasons. Knowing safety essentials is a priority. When necessary, you can always consult a professional aromatherapist for help. Following are my recommendations for using essential oils safely:

CONSIDER SPECIAL NEEDS. Use appropriate caution when using essential oils with infants, children, pregnant women, and older adults. These groups may be much more sensitive to the effects of essential oils than a typical adult. The remedies in this book are specially designed for pregnant women and are grouped according to whether they're used during pregnancy, labor, or the postpartum period. Use remedies only during the time period for which they're recommended.

AVOID MUCOUS MEMBRANES. Don't use any essential oils that are not diluted on or around the genitals and keep all oils away from the eyes, mouth, and nasal passages.

AVOID INTERNAL USE. Don't take essential oils internally; that is, don't ingest them. Although some companies that sell essential oils advocate that the oils be taken internally, this practice has not been proved to be safe. I never recommend that essential oils be ingested.

PATCH TEST

When I work with aromatherapy clients, I always suggest doing a patch test before using any essential oil. The simple instructions for doing a patch test on yourself follow:

- Apply 1 to 2 drops of the diluted essential oil inside the crease of your elbow.
- Cover the area with a bandage and keep it dry for 24 hours. Do not wash the area.
- If irritation, itching, redness, or swelling occurs, this essential oil may not be the one for you.
- Remember that if the essential oil doesn't cause a reaction for you, it may for someone else.

ALWAYS MIX WITH A CARRIER OIL. I've been using essential oils for over twenty-five years, and I never apply essential oils neat, or without dilution. I always use a carrier oil because I'm never sure how an essential oil will act or react with any person, even me, and using a carrier oil reduces the risk of a negative reaction. A carrier oil can be any nut, seed, or vegetable oil (see box, page 14).

BE AWARE OF THE POTENTIAL FOR ALLERGIES AND SENSITIVITIES. Essential oils can cause an allergic reaction or sensitivity. There are several steps you can take to prevent a reaction: never use undiluted essential oils, do a patch test (see box, above), and alternate the essential oils you use so that a sensitivity doesn't develop.

If an allergic reaction occurs when an essential oil is used topically, remove as much of it as you can by wiping the skin with a cloth soaked in milk or vegetable oil. The essential oil will bond with the fat in the milk or oil. Follow that with a thorough washing or shower.

LESS IS MORE. Although people tend to think that more of a good thing can only be better, this is not the case when working with essential oils. In fact, the opposite is true; it's always best to use the smallest effective amount. For example, if the recommended dosage is five drops, see if you get the same results with just two drops. Don't make a formula any stronger than necessary. And keep in mind that pregnant women are super-smellers, so following the less-is-more maxim is even more important for this population.

PAY ATTENTION TO IRRITATION. If irritation occurs, stop using the essential oil. Irritation can include feeling irritable or can refer to what's happening on the skin, such as contact dermatitis, hives, a rash, or redness. Irritation can occur with any application; if a diffused essential oil puts you in a bad mood, that's a negative reaction and reason to stop using that essential oil.

KEEP AWAY FROM FLAMES. Remember that essential oils are flammable. Use caution when using near an open flame, such as a candle diffuser.

STORING ESSENTIAL OILS

Since essential oils can be expensive, it's important to store them with care so they last. Here are some simple storage guidelines:

PROPER CONTAINERS. Make sure all essential oils are sold and stored in dark bottles with tightly sealed caps. Droppers should never be left on the bottles to function as caps during storage.

PROPER STORAGE. Store all essential oils in a cool, dark place. Exposure to direct sunlight in particular or any light in general will speed up oxidation and break down the essential oil.

SHELF LIFE. Most essential oils have a shelf life of two years. Some, such as citrus oils, keep for only one year. Pine and tea tree oil keep for about eighteen months. Patchouli and sandalwood keep a good bit longer than most, up to four years.

MIXING. Always mix essential oils with carrier oils (see box, page 14) in glass bottles or jars or porcelain or aluminum bottles (aluminum bottles must have a phenolic lining). Never use plastic because essential oils can degrade it.

After putting the carrier oil in the bottle, use a dropper to add the essential oil or oils. I recommend that you use a separate dropper for every essential oil. Make sure you draw the essential oil only into the glass stem and not into the dropper's bulb. The bulb is rubber, and it will degrade and break down if exposed to essential oils over a prolonged period.

CLEANING. Use vodka or another alcohol to clean the droppers. Draw the vodka into the dropper and allow it to soak in the dropper. Alternatively, take the bulb off the stem and let both pieces soak in white vinegar before rinsing with boiling water to sterilize.

BLENDING ESSENTIAL OILS: THE BASICS

If one essential oil is good, combining two or more can be better. Blend essential oils for their fragrance or therapeutic value, or both. Always follow safety tips (see pages 10 to 12) when blending oils and creating aromatherapy applications. Basic methods for creating aromatherapy

The scent of a blend of essential oils changes over time. This is because different essential oils have varying evaporation rates. As the essential oils in the blend evaporate, the odor changes to reflect the aromas of the remaining oil or oils:

- Top notes evaporate in one to two hours. Top notes tend to be the primary or most noticeable scent you detect in a blend.
- Middle notes are slightly heavier and evaporate in two to four hours. These are often herbaceous scents.
- Base notes take longer to evaporate—sometimes several days.

products are described in chapter 5, "Making Your Own Aromatherapy and Herbal Remedies," pages 77 to 87.

BALANCING A BLEND

The trick to balancing a blend of essential oils is to know which families get along. That is, essential oils can be characterized into broad groups, or families, based on their aroma types. Essential oils in the same family typically blend well together. The following list shows which families blend well with each other:

- Exotic and spicy scents blend well with citrusy and floral scents.
- Flowery scents blend well with citrusy, spicy, and woodsy scents.
- Minty scents blend well with citrusy, earthy, herbaceous, and woodsy scents.
- Woodsy and outdoorsy scents generally blend well with all other families.

It's easy to experiment with blending. Take a few drops of three different essential oils, smell each one separately, and then mix them together. How does the combination differ from the original essential oils? How does the scent change over time as the essential oils begin to evaporate? Several hours can make quite a difference in the scent of any essential oil blend. (See "Top, Middle, and Base Notes," above.)

The following is a common grouping of essential oil families:

CITRUSY. Citrusy oils are often top notes, evaporate pretty quickly, and blend well with most scents. The most popular citrus essential oils are grapefruit, lemon, lemon balm, lime, mandarin, orange, sweet orange, and tangerine.

To be used safely, essential oils must first be mixed with carrier oils. Carrier oils are common oils made from nuts, seeds, and vegetables. Apricot kernel oil, olive oil, and sweet almond oil are some examples.

In some of my remedies, I suggest specific carrier oils, but most often I don't, letting it be your choice. Sometimes I choose a carrier oil based on the season. For example, in the winter I might use a thicker oil, such as olive oil or warmed coconut oil; in the summer, I might use a lighter oil, such as apricot kernel oil or grapeseed oil.

Note: Carrier oils are added only after the essential oils are mixed and when you're ready to use the blend.

EARTHY. Earthy scents, which are typically base notes, bring to mind fresh air, earth, and water. These include patchouli and vetiver.

EXOTIC. Typically middle and base notes, exotic essential oils are all lovely and include ginger, patchouli, sandalwood, and ylang-ylang.

FLOWERY. Floral scents are often top notes or middle notes. These include jasmine, lavender, neroli, palmarosa, rose, and ylang-ylang.

HERBACEOUS. Made from herbs, these essential oils have a distinctively "green" scent and include basil, clary sage, and hyssop.

MEDICINAL OR CAMPHOROUS. Usually top and middle notes, these essential oils include eucalyptus and tea tree.

MINTY. The mint family is among the most familiar essential oils and includes lavender, peppermint, and spearmint. These tend to be top and middle notes.

SPICY. Warm, often exotic, and reminiscent of certain kitchen spices, these scents include allspice, cardamom, cassia, and clove.

WOODSY. Woodsy essential oils are middle or base notes and evoke thoughts of nature and the outdoors. These include cedarwood, cypress, pine, and spruce. Note that while cypress essential oil is particularly useful during the postpartum period, it is not recommended for use during pregnancy.

STOCKING UP ON THE ESSENTIALS

In addition to the essential oils themselves, only a few pieces of equipment and ingredients are needed to make aromatherapy blends. Most are items that you may already have at home, and all are inexpensive.

CARRIER OILS. Used in liniments, massage oils, and other topical applications, carrier oils are used to "carry" the essential oil. Carrier oils can be any nut, seed, or vegetable oil (see box, opposite page).

LIQUIDS. Used in liniments, sprays, and toners, various liquids can be added to essential oils. These include water, witch hazel, or a food-grade alcohol, such as vodka.

DROPPER BOTTLES OR GLASS JARS WITH LIDS. Essential oils are volatile and begin to evaporate upon contact with the air, so it's advisable to immediately put the cap or lid on the bottle or jar after putting in the essential oils. Add a few drops at a time to the bottle, put on the cap, and gently swish the essential oils to mix.

DROPPERS OR PIPETTES. Droppers are slender glass tubes that have a rubber bulb at one end. They're used for transferring liquids or essential oils to a bottle or jar. Pipettes are thin glass tubes that may incorporate a glass bulb at one end; they also can be used for this purpose. At about ten cents apiece, pipettes are affordable and can be reused when cleaned properly. Droppers are more expensive but are also reusable when cleaned properly.

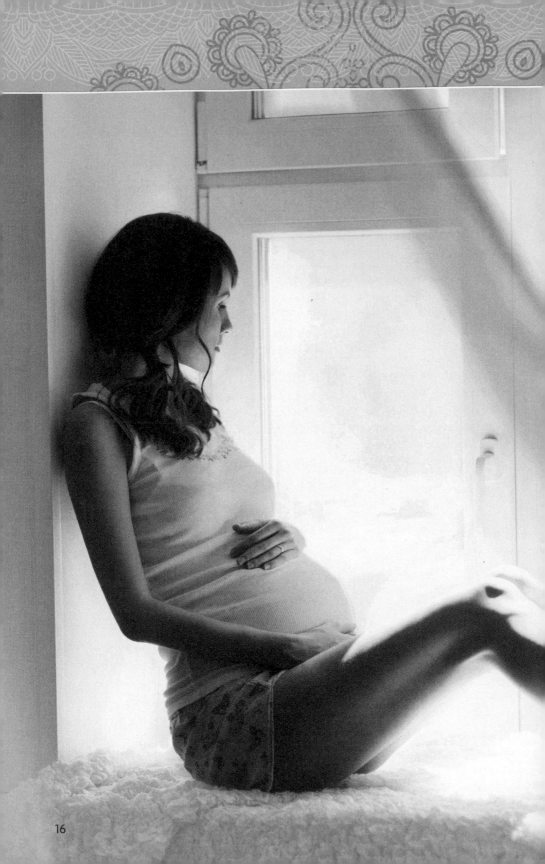

Essential Oils for Pregnancy, Labor, and Breastfeeding

Essential oils come from various sources; accordingly, they feature an array of different scents and offer a range of therapeutic effects. This chapter lists some common essential oils that are used in aromatherapy. The first list features essential oils that are safe to use during pregnancy, birth, and breastfeeding and includes short descriptions of their attributes and uses. Equally important are the two following lists, which highlight essential oils that are *not* safe to use during pregnancy (see page 22) and those that are not safe to use in general (see page 23).

Note that the information in this chapter applies only to aromatherapy and essential oils. Some of the same plants may be available in other forms (such as dried flowers or leaves) that are used in herbalism, and recommendations for their use may differ. See chapter 4, "Herbs for Pregnancy, Labor, and Breastfeeding," pages 49 to 75, for lists that apply to herbs, including those that are used in herbal remedies and culinary herbs that are used in food preparation.

The following lists contain scientific terms that may be unfamiliar. For example, "abortifacient" is a word used to refer to essential oils that can cause contractions and abortions. The Glossary (see page 171) supplies definitions for many of the terms used in this chapter.

ESSENTIAL OILS THAT ARE SAFE FOR USE

Bergamot *(Citrus bergamia)*

Fresh and citrusy, bergamot essential oil lifts a dark mood and eases feelings of depression. It blends well with many oils, especially Roman chamomile and all citrus oils.

Black pepper *(Piper nigrum)*

Used in topical applications, black pepper essential oil is included in blends designed to relieve sore muscles, painful varicose veins, and muscular tension. It's good for promoting regional circulation.

Chamomile, Roman *(Anthemis nobilis)*

Long used for skin and wound care, Roman chamomile essential oil is beneficial in treating bruises, insect bites, psoriasis, sprains, and swelling. Because it's relaxing and relieves spasms, it's also helpful in treating muscle and nerve pain. For example, applying a chamomile compress can provide relief from pain. If Roman chamomile essential oil is not available, German chamomile or chamomile essential oil can be used instead, because these oils share similar properties.

Cypress *(Cupressus sempervirens)*

Noted for its ability to heal wounds, soothe sore muscles, and relieve cramping, cypress essential oil has a number of beneficial properties. It's antibacterial, anti-inflammatory, and antiseptic; it works well as a deodorant, expectorant, sedative, and tonic.

CONTRAINDICATIONS: Although cypress essential oil is not safe to use during pregnancy, it can be used safely during the postpartum period.

Eucalyptus *(Eucalyptus radiata; Eucalyptus globulus)*

Long used as a therapy for respiratory ailments, eucalyptus is a great essential oil for treating colds, congestion, flu, and sinus problems, including infections. It's antibacterial, antifungal, and antiseptic; it also relieves pain and spasms. In addition, it's a good treatment for wounds, although it can cause skin irritation.

Frankincense *(Boswellia carteri)*

Soothing and relaxing, frankincense essential oil is popular for relieving anxiety and stress. It can be diffused or made into a compress. As an expectorant, it's valuable in treating asthma and bronchitis. Used topically in a compress, lotion, or massage oil, it's an effective chest rub and antiseptic; it's also good for treating rheumatism and scars.

Geranium (Pelargonium graveolens)

Geranium essential oil is frequently included in blends designed to alleviate depression or lift a dark mood. In addition, many people love the regenerative properties this oil offers in skin-care formulas. Recent research also has shown this oil's potential in treating and managing pain. For example, blended with a carrier oil or mixed into a salve, geranium essential oil can be helpful in treating nerve pain, neuropathy, and shingles.

CONTRAINDICATIONS: Although geranium essential oil is not safe to use during pregnancy, it can be used safely during the postpartum period.

Grapefruit (Citrus paradisi)

Light and refreshing, grapefruit essential oil is one of my favorites. It's great for treating anxiety, irritability, and stress, especially during times of hormonal upheaval and exhaustion—or when a lift in spirits is needed. It's antibacterial, antiseptic, astringent, restorative, and stimulating; it also aids depression and digestion.

Lavender (Lavandula angustifolia)

Lavender essential oil is beloved for its skin-healing properties in addition to its many other uses. In a diffuser blend, it can promote a calm, relaxing environment and lessen stress; it even relaxes and soothes infants. It's also earned a place in any first-aid kit because it can treat cuts and scrapes, insect bites, sore muscles, and sunburn. In addition, it's helpful in treating stress and tension. For example, a lavender compress can be used to relieve a headache, muscle pain, stress, and sunburn.

Lavender is considered one of the safest essential oils on the market. Some sources say it's okay to use lavender essential oil neat, or without dilution; however, to prevent reactions, I recommend that lavender essential oil always be diluted. Sensitivity can occur suddenly or after long-term use, and mixing lavender with a carrier oil can help prevent this.

Lemon (Citrus limon)

A staple in many homes, lemon essential oil is used in a variety of household applications. It's an effective antifungal.

Mandarin (Citrus reticulata)

Good at promoting sleep and relaxation and relieving insomnia and stress, mandarin essential oil is also excellent when you're feeling tired and sluggish. In addition, it's beneficial for skin issues, such as acne, aging skin, dull skin, oily skin, and scars.

Neroli *(Citrus aurantium)*

Traditionally used to treat depression, stress, and other types of emotional upheaval, neroli essential oil is also beneficial for skin issues, including mature skin and stretch marks, and is often found in skin creams and oils. Obtained from orange blossoms, this essential oil is coveted for its ability to mix well with almost all other essential oils.

Niaouli *(Melaleuca viridiflora)*

Niaouli essential oil is beneficial for relaxing muscles and alleviating tension. It makes a wonderful addition to a soothing bath.

Patchouli *(Pogostemon cablin)*

Sometimes called the "hippie oil" and often remembered as the scent of the 1960s, patchouli essential oil is an excellent base for an oil blend. Over time, its scent improves, its color changes, and it becomes richer.

Pine *(Pinus sylvestris)*

We all know the scent of pine. Refreshing and invigorating, it's in the air and in our cleaning products. In fact, the smell of pine is associated with a fresh and clean house. Used in inhalation therapy, pine essential oil helps clear the sinuses. When included in a massage oil, it's effective in treating acute joint pain.

Roman chamomile (SEE CHAMOMILE, ROMAN, PAGE 18)

Rose *(Rosa damascena)*

The delicate scent of rose is one of the most familiar in the world, and it's been valued for its sedative and aphrodisiac effects since the beginning of time. Rose essential oil is often found in facial oils and creams because it's both antibacterial and antiseptic.

Rose hip seed oil *(Rosa canina)*

Although rose hip seed oil is not a true essential oil, it can be found where essential oils are sold. With skin-rejuvenating attributes, rose hip seed oil is a safe and natural solution to repair the skin's surface. It is an excellent ingredient for stretch-mark remedies, and it also restores skin's elasticity and protects against sun and pollution.

Rosemary *(Rosmarinus officinalis)*

A versatile tool in any first-aid kit, rosemary essential oil is antimicrobial, making it an excellent treatment for cuts and scrapes. In addition, it clears congestion and is useful for treating headaches in general and migraines in particular. A good way to treat a headache is to combine a few drops of rosemary essential oil with a carrier oil (see box, page 14) and massage this mixture into the temples. In addition, research has shown that the scent of rosemary essential oil can improve cognitive performance as well as mood.

CONTRAINDICATIONS: Although rosemary essential oil is not safe to use during pregnancy, it can be used safely during the postpartum period.

Rosewood *(Aniba rosaeodora)*

Known for its uplifting effect, rosewood essential oil is stimulating, relieves depression, and acts as an aphrodisiac. It's also a good oil to use on mature skin. Rosewood essential oil is antiseptic, bactericidal, deodorizing, and insecticidal.

St. John's wort oil *(Hypericum perforatum)*

Sold as an infusion of St. John's wort flowers in a carrier oil (see box, page 14), this oil can be purchased or made at home (see the method for making infused oils, page 81). St. John's wort oil has been found to be beneficial in treating muscle aches and pains and back pain. Offering relief from inflammation, this soothing oil also acts as a wound-healing agent.

Sandalwood *(Santalum album)*

Sandalwood essential oil is one of my favorites. It is, in a word, exotic. I often suggest sandalwood essential oil for clients who want to relax and "get in the mood." If it succeeds in helping you make a baby, this essential oil can relieve the backache that occurs during pregnancy. It also relieves anxiety, headache, and skin flare-ups.

Some sandalwood is not ethically or sustainably harvested. When purchasing sandalwood essential oil, make sure it comes from a sustainable source. See Suppliers (page 173) for reputable sources.

Sweet orange *(Citrus sinensis)*

Sweet orange essential oil is a light oil that is used in many everyday items, including air fresheners, cleaning products, and laundry soaps. Therapeutically, it alleviates feelings of anxiety and stress. For example, it's effective for treating sadness and depression, including postpartum depression.

Tangerine *(Citrus reticulata)*

I love the smell of citrus essential oils and especially tangerine. It has an uplifting effect for people who are feeling sluggish or worn down.

This essential oil is antiseptic, relieves spasms, and is a sedative; for example, it's beneficial for stress and insomnia.

Tea tree (Melaleuca alternifolia)

Tea tree is an extremely popular essential oil, with good reason; it's effective in addressing a wide range of issues. If you are pregnant and experience bacterial vaginosis (see page 98), you can add a drop or two to a cup of water and soak a tampon in that solution before inserting it. Or add a drop or two to a sitz bath. In addition, tea tree essential oil can be used to treat acne, athlete's foot, candida, chicken pox, colds, cold sores, cuts and scrapes, flu, headaches, insect bites, and itchiness. It also works as a decongestant, deodorant, and expectorant. All this is possible because this versatile oil is analgesic, antibacterial, antifungal, anti-inflammatory, antimicrobial, antiseptic, antiviral, fungicidal, and insecticidal.

Vetiver (Vetiveria zizanoides)

With its mellow and slightly earthy scent, vetiver essential oil is known for its anti-inflammatory, antiseptic, aphrodisiac, and sedative actions. This oil has a grounding and calming effect for many people. In addition, it's beneficial for dry skin, sore joints, and sore muscles.

Ylang-ylang (Cananga odorata)

Ylang-ylang essential oil is considered relaxing, and it's useful for hormonal mood swings associated with premenstrual syndrome and menopause. In a diffuser blend, this essential oil can assist with feelings of angst, anxiety, and irritability. Also effective against depression, it's found in many antidepressant blends.

ESSENTIAL OILS TO AVOID DURING PREGNANCY

The following essential oils should be avoided during pregnancy. Some stimulate abortion, blood flow, or contractions; all are potentially dangerous to the mother, the baby, or both.

Although these essential oils should be avoided during pregnancy, some are safe to use during the postpartum period, and these are marked with asterisks. Note too that none of these essential oils should be confused with herbs used in herbal remedies (see pages 50 to 68) or culinary herbs used in food preparation (see page 75).

Anise (Pimpinella anisum)	Cypress (Cupressus sempervirens)*
Blue tansy (Tanacetum annuum)	Davana (Artemisia pallens)
Clove (Eugenia caryophyllata)	Geranium (Pelargonium graveolens)*

Holy basil (*Ocimum gratissimum; Ocimum tenuiflorum*)

Juniper (*Juniperus communis*)

Kanuka (*Leptospermum ericoides*)

Lavandin (*Lavandula hybrida*)

Linden blossom (*Tilia vulgaris*)

Marjoram (*Origanum majorana*)

Myrrh (*Commiphora myrrha*)

Oakmoss (*Evernia prunastri*)

Oregano (*Origanum vulgare*)

Palo santo (*Bursera graveolens*)

Peru balsam (*Myroxylon pereirae*)

Ravensara (*Ravensara aromatica*)

Rose geranium (*Pelargonium roseum*)

Rosemary (*Rosmarinus officinalis*)*

Sage or Dalmatian sage (*Salvia officinalis*)

Saro or mandravasarotra (*Cinnamosma fragrans*)

Spanish sage (*Salvia lavandulaefolia*)

ESSENTIAL OILS TO AVOID IN GENERAL

The following essential oils are known to be unsafe for anyone, pregnant or otherwise, and trained aromatherapists avoid them. Although many sources don't say why these essential oils should not be used, I've included what information I can. In most cases, there are safe alternatives to any of the following essential oils.

Ajowan (*Trachyspermum copticum*)

Because ajowan essential oil has a high thymol content, which can cause contractions, it should be avoided during pregnancy. Undiluted, this essential oil irritates the skin and mucous membranes.

Almond, bitter (*Prunus dulcis* var. *amara*)

Bitter almond essential oil should never be used therapeutically because it contains hydrocyanic acid, which is poisonous.

Arnica (*Arnica montana*)

Arnica essential oil is unsafe to use during pregnancy; however, an infused oil or a homeopathic remedy made from arnica flowers can be used, as can over-the-counter formulations of arnica cream or gel.

Atlas cedarwood (*Cedrus atlantica*)

Atlas cedarwood essential oil is a potential abortifacient.

Basil (*Ocimum basilicum*)

Basil essential oil should be used sparingly and with caution. Higher doses of this oil may be carcinogenic, particularly when made with basil that contains a significant amount of methyl chavicol, which has psychoactive effects. Basil essential oil should not be used by anyone with liver problems.

Bay *(Pimenta racemosa)*

Bay essential oil can be problematic for individuals with liver issues.

Bay laurel *(Laurus nobilis)*

Bay laurel essential oil can cause contact dermatitis.

Birch, sweet *(Betula lenta)*

The main constituent of sweet birch essential oil is methyl salicylate, the active ingredient in aspirin, and this oil is especially problematic for anyone who is sensitive or allergic to aspirin. It should be avoided by women who are pregnant or breastfeeding. It's also not safe for children, older adults, and individuals who have liver problems, are on blood-thinning medication, or have epilepsy or seizures.

Bitter almond (SEE ALMOND, BITTER, PAGE 23)

Boldo *(Peumus boldus)*

Boldo essential oil contains ascaridole, which is considered highly toxic and often referred to as an abortifacient. According to my research, no one in the aromatherapy community considers this oil to be safe.

Broom, Spanish *(Spartium junceum)*

Spanish broom essential oil is considered toxic according to most sources. Avoid this essential oil for all uses in aromatherapy.

Brown camphor (SEE CAMPHOR, BROWN, BELOW)

Calamus *(Acorus calamus var. angustatus)*

Calamus is a newer essential oil and not enough research has been done regarding its safety. To date, many sources cite it as unsafe for use in aromatherapy.

Camphor, brown *(Cinnamomum camphora)* and Camphor, yellow *(Cinnamomum camphora)*

Some sources say that camphor essential oil has no contraindications for human use, and others state it is toxic and unsafe. Animal studies show that it can have toxic effects on the embryo.

Cedarwood, Atlas (SEE PAGE 23)

Cedarwood, Virginia *(Juniperus virginiana)*

Most aromatherapy books say that cedarwood essential oil is not safe to use during pregnancy, although some sources say there is little evidence to indicate whether it is safe or not.

Clary sage *(Salvia sclarea)*

Although clary sage essential oil is not safe to use during pregnancy, it can safely be used during labor.

Deertongue *(Carphephorus odoratissimus)*

Not a lot of information is available about deertongue essential oil, but when it's discussed, it's described as toxic.

Elemi *(Canarium luzonicum)*

Elemi essential oil is considered a potential carcinogen.

Fennel *(Foeniculum vulgare)*

Fennel essential oil can be potentially narcotic if used in large doses.

Garlic *(Allium sativum)*

Garlic essential oil can cause severe skin irritation. In some people, it can trigger breathing problems.

Horseradish *(Armoracia rusticana)*

Horseradish oil contains allyl isothiocyanate and is known to irritate the skin, eyes, nose, and mucous membranes.

Hyssop *(Hyssopus officinalis)*

Hyssop essential oil has been linked to convulsions and seizures. It also is reported to cause vomiting. These side effects are more likely when high doses are used.

Jaborandi *(Pilocarpus jaborandi)*

Jaborandi essential oil can cause a general ill feeling and a host of other side effects, including diarrhea, respiratory distress, vision disturbances, and vomiting.

Jasmine *(Jasminum grandiflorum)*

Because jasmine essential oil can cause strong contractions, it should be used only when labor is already under way. This oil should never be used to stimulate labor.

May chang (Litsea cubeba)

May chang essential oil can cause glaucoma and skin damage or disease.

Melilot (Melilotus officinalis)

Melilot essential oil is known to irritate the skin and is thought to contain the chemical coumarin, a compound used in making anticoagulants. Individuals taking blood thinners should avoid this oil until more information is known.

Mugwort (Artemisia vulgaris)

Mugwort essential oil contains the potentially dangerous neurotoxin thujone and is a potential abortifacient.

Mustard (Brassica nigra)

Mustard oil contains allyl isothiocyanate and is a known irritant to the skin, eyes, nose, and mucous membranes.

Nutmeg (Myristica fragrans)

Nutmeg essential oil can cause nausea and increase the heart rate (tachycardia).

Onion (Allium cepa)

Onion oil can cause contact irritation, dizziness, and nausea.

Parsley (Petroselinum sativum)

Parsley essential oil is considered an abortifacient.

Pennyroyal (Mentha pulegium)

Pennyroyal essential oil is an abortifacient. It can also cause acute liver and lung damage, even in small doses. If ingested in large doses, this oil can cause death.

Peppermint (Mentha piperata)

Although peppermint essential oil should generally be avoided during pregnancy, a small amount can safely be inhaled to prevent dizziness, fainting, or nausea. A gentler alternative is spearmint essential oil.

Rue (Ruta graveolens)

Rue essential oil can burn and irritate the skin.

Sassafras *(Sassafras albidum)*

Potentially lethal, sassafras essential oil is never safe to use.

Spanish broom (SEE BROOM, SPANISH, PAGE 24)

Star anise *(Illicium verum)*

Star anise essential oil should not be used because it slows circulation.

Sweet birch (SEE BIRCH, SWEET, PAGE 24)

Tansy *(Tanacetum vulgare)*

Tansy essential oil can cause convulsions, vomiting, and uterine bleeding. It can be fatal as the result of respiratory arrest and organ failure.

Thuja *(Thuja occidentalis)*

Thuja essential oil can cause abortion or miscarriage.

Thyme *(Thymus vulgaris)*

Thyme essential oil can elevate blood pressure.

Virginia cedarwood (SEE CEDARWOOD, VIRGINIA, PAGE 25)

Wintergreen *(Gaultheria procumbens)*

Wintergreen essential oil can be fatal if ingested.

Wormseed *(Chenopodium ambrosioides var. anthelminticum)*

Wormseed oil should not be used in aromatherapy. In addition, the oil may explode when heated or treated with acids.

Wormwood *(Artemisia absinthium)*

Wormwood essential oil contains an extremely high amount of thujone, which can be a convulsant and neurotoxin.

Yarrow *(Achillea millefolium)*

Yarrow essential oil is considered a neurotoxin.

Yellow camphor (SEE CAMPHOR, YELLOW, PAGE 24)

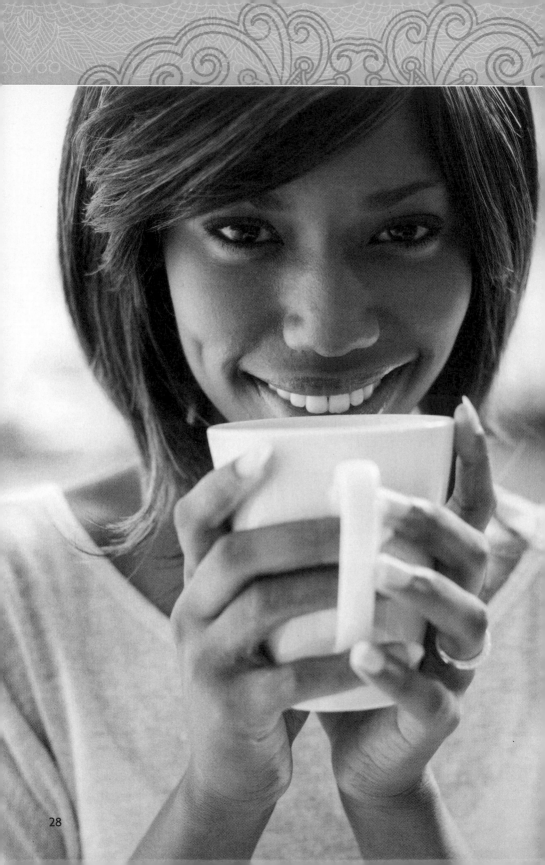

CHAPTER 3

Introduction to Herbal Remedies

Almost every midwife I know works with herbs on some level, and many other professionals who provide care to pregnant women also use herbal remedies, which are sometimes called herbals. Like aromatherapy, which relies on essential oils derived from plants, herbalism is based on the ancient practice of using plants as medicine. However, whereas essential oils can only be used externally through topical applications and inhalations, herbal remedies can be used topically or ingested. In herbalism, remedies that are ingested are said to be taken internally. Herbs are used in compresses, liniments, and salves, much the way essential oils are used; all of these remedies are used topically. An example of an herbal that is taken internally is a cup of tea, which can be infused from fresh or dried flowers, leaves, roots, or a combination of these. Many varieties of ready-made herbal teas are available in easy-to-use tea bags. Chances are, you have a box of these teas in your pantry right now. Other herbals, such as extracts and tinctures, are more concentrated and are taken by the dropperful or teaspoonful. Finally, one of the most common uses of herbs is in food preparation; we routinely encounter herbs in salads and other dishes, which just goes to show how safe herbal use is, even during pregnancy.

During the past twenty years in the United States, increasing public dissatisfaction with the cost, questionable safety, and lack of effectiveness of prescription medications, combined with an interest in returning to natural remedies, has led to a phenomenal resurgence in the use of herbal medicines. A 2001 study found that almost 70 percent of Americans have used at least one form of alternative therapy in their lifetimes, making this "unconventional" medical approach one of the fastest-growing categories of American health care. I know from my ever-growing student population that not just one demographic exists for people interested in herbalism and aromatherapy. These days, people from all walks of life are looking into these increasingly conventional therapies.

The World Health Organization has estimated that more than 80 percent of the world's population depends on herbal medicines for some measure of their primary health care. In Germany and Switzerland, between six hundred and seven hundred plant-based medicines are available and are prescribed by approximately 70 percent of physicians. In many parts of Europe, herbals are blended and compounded in the same apothecary shops where prescription medications are sold.

Some sources state that up to 90 percent of midwives work with herbals and that up to 52 percent of all women in Canada use herbal remedies during pregnancy. In the United States it is difficult to find accurate usage rates. Some sources say 10 percent, and others estimate much higher rates. This disparity is rooted, in part, by patients' fear of telling their doctors they are using herbs or any other alternative therapy. Many doctors do not know much about herbs, but that doesn't mean they aren't interested in supporting your choices or aren't willing to learn. Letting your doctor or midwife know what you want in your care plan is essential.

One of the greatest benefits of herbal medicine for families is that it is readily available to all who choose to use it. Herbs and herbal products are readily available at practically any retail outlet—at natural food stores, supermarkets, drugstores, and even your gas station convenience store. This availability is a good thing, but it can be a bad thing if you don't know the quality and content of what you're buying. The advantage of a book like this one is that it allows you to make your own herbal remedies, which is relatively easy to do once you've found reliable sources for fresh and dry ingredients (see Suppliers, page 173).

I like to think of herbal medicine as a natural approach. During the last five thousand years, people have used different methods to treat health disorders, and many have been plant-based medicinal preparations. The intelligence and practicality of early herbalists has brought us to where we are today, both in herbal and traditional medicine. Those pioneers have helped us recognize that we are part of nature, not separate from it, and that we can find what we need in and from nature.

Through a basic process of experimentation, these incredible people began to remember, record, and collect information and remedies they then handed down to the next generation. Thanks to their efforts, we have learned which plants nourish a pregnant woman, for example, or soothe a cough.

Throughout much of history, herbalism was not the practice we think of today. Rather, it was hands-on remedy-making, based on healing methods not limited by definitions or governmental regulatory bodies. Its history is tightly intertwined with that of modern medicine and midwifery (see "An Herbal Timeline," below). Many of the first herbalists were women, mothers, and midwives. Up until about one hundred years ago, the woman of the house made most of her family's medicine, a tradition that is coming back into vogue as parents again take charge of their family's health. In part, the technology that powers our information age also is driving this trend. You can find blogs about moms who are fitting the old ways into their modern lives.

AN HERBAL TIMELINE

Herbal medicine was the people's medicine—it grew wherever they were. The practice of herbal medicine has been documented in ancient African, Chinese, Greek, Indian, Native American, Roman, and Tibetan cultures for thousands of years. Ultimately, the search for herbs led European explorers to seek and discover India and, by proxy, North America.

In Shanidar Cave in Iraq, pollen samples were found with human remains, indicating that Neanderthals who lived between 80,000 and 60,000 BP had been treated with herbal medicine. Remedies used at the time included bachelor's button, cornflower, grape hyacinth, hollyhock, yarrow, and other herbs.

Herbal medicine was used during the New Stone Age (8000–5000 BCE), when women gathered and men hunted. As the gatherers ventured forth for food each day, they took into account what was available and useful in their natural surroundings. Women practiced herbalism daily and were always on the lookout for what was growing and when it was at its peak of potency and nutrition.

The world's oldest surviving medical document, *Ebers Papyrus*, dates to 2000 BCE and lists medicinal prescriptions that have greatly influenced even today's modern medicine. In the ancient libraries of the Achaemenid Dynasty (550–330 BCE), also known as the Persian Empire, there are texts containing lists of plants, herbs, and other substances used for medicinal purposes.

Although we know from recorded European history that herbal medicine was documented at the time of the Roman invasions, we also have anthropological evidence that herbs were used by the ancient Celts. Soutra Aisle, on the Scottish border, is believed to have been the site of one of the largest hospitals in the region during medieval times and dates from 1164 CE. Evidence of the use of hemlock, opium poppy, and other common herbs of the time has been unearthed there. An extremely important Welsh text, *The Red Book of Hergest* (circa 1425), described more than five hundred ways to use two hundred herbs. Herbs became such an important tool for healing that, in 1542, King Henry VIII signed a charter ensuring herbalists the right to practice.

During the battles of World War I, herbs were used for treating burns, preventing infections, and as antiseptics. In 1941, the British government appealed to civilians to collect, grow, and identify herbs to be made into medicine. Now, British herbalists practice and are protected under the 1968 Medicines Act.

In the Americas, natives had used medicinal herbs for a thousand years before the Europeans arrived. They had accumulated a vast store of botanical and medical knowledge, a fact that surprised many European explorers. When the Europeans returned home, they took many native plants and Native American remedies. These became part of European herbal literature and practice.

Today, many primitive tribes retain an expert knowledge of medicinal plants and their uses, and their plant "databases" can number into the hundreds. Contemporary herbalists have access to a great many texts by the elders of all nations. The world has a huge pharmacopoeia that is the basis for most of our modern pharmaceuticals.

In addition, throughout history almost every culture has combined some aspect of spirituality, from a simple prayer to a shamanistic ritual, with healing. Healers have traditionally called upon the spiritual world to assist them in their work, and many continue to do so today.

USING HERBS SAFELY

Because of herbal medicine's long history, we have had enough time to learn which plants and remedies are tried and true, what to use when, and which to avoid. Like other herbalists, I draw on these traditions when formulating remedies. When treating expectant mothers, I can confidently say herbal remedies are generally safe. However, as is the case for any type of medical therapy, there are guidelines that must be followed, precautions that should be taken, and knowledge that should be gained before the treatment is under way.

There's so much more involved in the issue of herbal safety than whether the herbs themselves are intrinsically harmless. In addition, each phase—pregnancy, labor and delivery, and the postpartum period and breastfeeding—requires special consideration. Accordingly, the remedies in this book are divided into three chapters that cover each period.

You always have the option to enlist the help of a professional herbalist when you are expecting. Whether or not you decide to do so, if you are considering the use of herbal remedies, I urge you to educate yourself; if possible, do so before you become pregnant. Unfortunately, most of the time when we are confronted with decisions about our health, we are already overcome with worry, which makes it difficult to gather new information on which to base our actions.

My recommendation is to do two things. First, familiarize yourself with pregnancy: Learn about nutrition and issues common during pregnancy. Get to know what the body goes through or might go through so that when you become familiar with herbs you'll recognize which ones you'll need to treat the problem. Next, learn about herbs and herbal medicine. Take classes. Peruse websites and books: read, read, read.

HERBAL APPLICATIONS

Some herbal applications are designed to be taken internally. These include decoctions, infusions, extracts, tinctures, syrups, and lozenges. Like aromatherapy applications, other herbal applications are used externally. These include compresses, poultices, and plasters; liniments; and salves. Following are brief descriptions of these types of remedies. For information about how each is made, see chapter 5, "Making Your Own Aromatherapy and Herbal Remedies," pages 77 to 87.

Decoctions

A decoction is the concentrated liquor that remains after heating or boiling down an herb, specifically the more tenacious parts of the plant, such as the bark, nuts, or roots, or a combination.

Infusions and Teas

An infusion is a remedy made by soaking plant parts or dried herbs in a liquid. Herbal tea is the most well-known and popular herbal infusion, requiring only the herbs and boiled water. Herbs can also be infused in oil.

Extracts and Tinctures

Tinctures and extracts are made by extracting the active properties of the herb in food-grade alcohol. A tincture is traditionally a diluted extract. Unfortunately, the terms "extract" and "tincture" are often interchanged and misused these days. Both can be purchased or made at home. When shopping, read the label carefully to make sure you are buying what you think you are buying.

Lozenges

Lozenges, or pastilles, are easy-to-make, portable herbal preparations, mainly used to help aid digestion, alleviate sore throats, calm coughs, and freshen breath. Lozenges are great to have in the birth room instead of hard candy to moisten your mouth.

Syrups

Whether store-bought or homemade, medicinal syrups, such as cough syrups, are made from herbs. During pregnancy, syrups can help provide nutritional support.

Compresses, Poultices, and Plasters

Used topically, often to decrease pain and swelling, a compress is made by soaking a piece of cloth in a cold or warm infusion and applying it to the affected area. A poultice, which is applied warm, is similar to a compress except that fresh herbs are used instead of an infusion. A plaster is similar to a poultice, but dried herbs are typically used.

Liniments

A liniment is an herbal extraction in a liquid, such as food-grade alcohol, oil, or vinegar, which is rubbed into the skin to treat arthritis, inflammations, sore muscles, and strains.

Salves

Salves are creams or emollients that provide barrier protection while carrying medicinal benefits. A salve is a mixture of an herb-infused oil with a hard wax, such as beeswax, candelilla wax, or coconut oil. When I was pregnant, I used salves all over my body. They soothed dry skin, prevented stretch marks, and kept my skin soft and nourished. Now that my children are grown, salves are still the primary tools in my medicine chest. Most of my family's aches and pains, bruises, cuts, scrapes, and strains are treated with salves. When buying prepared herbal salves, look for the appropriate herb, of course, but also make sure the remaining ingredients are ones you recognize and have names you can understand.

JUDGING HERBAL QUALITY

How can you judge the quality of an herb? The ultimate test for any herb is to use it in a remedy and gauge its potency and effectiveness. This is also the best way to evaluate whether or not to purchase from a particular supplier in the future. Whether you grow your own, purchase from a natural food store, harvest from the wild, or buy from a bulk supplier, consider the following when judging whether an herb will be effective:

- Fresh herbs should retain their fresh color, aroma, and taste. Their leaves and roots should look alive and healthy.
- Dried herbs should remain pretty much in their whole state. The flowers should look like flowers, the leaves like leaves, and so on.
- Dried herbs should not be mostly stems and dust. The more broken down the herb, the shorter its shelf life. Sift through the dried herb with your fingers and look at the color and texture.
- Dried herbs should smell and taste vibrant and fresh, not musty and old.

BUYING HERBS

Always buy organically grown herbs. Most large herb companies fumigate their plants because pests could wipe out their entire stock. Many companies also have begun to irradiate their herbs to kill pests. Buying herbs from a distributor who uses overseas suppliers increases your chances of getting irradiated products.

Using chemical-free herbs is as important as eating chemical-free foods, but not just for our personal health. When we choose organics, we promote sustainable farming and biodiversity, help decrease pollution, protect the soil and water, and make work safer for farmers and farm workers. Think how much better you will feel, not just physically but also emotionally, when you nourish your body and your family with clean, honorably produced herbs and food. When we make choices that protect our environment, we are also making choices that protect our bodies.

Buying locally supports your neighbors and smaller farms. Shop for organic herbs at your farmers' market, which is also a great place to get starter plants for your garden, vegetables, fruits, and herbs. Get to know the people who grow them. When I buy garlic or echinacea plants from the farmer down the road, I know I'm getting fresh and potent garlic and strong echinacea that will do their jobs in my remedies.

If you can't buy locally, seek out organic herbs and herbal products at natural food stores—usually in the bulk section—or from specialty retailers. Research your source. For a list of recommended online and mail-order suppliers, see pages 173 to 174.

GROWING YOUR OWN HERBS

Gardening books may feature elaborate herbal knot gardens that look complicated and intimidating, but the fact is, herbs are easy to grow. And they can be grown just about anywhere there is good soil, sunshine, and water (and maybe a little compost once in a while). You can grow herbs in a small plot in the yard; in a corner of your garden; or in pots on your porch, patio, or kitchen windowsill.

Basic information about growing herbs can be found in almost any gardening book. Alternatively, ask local gardeners and herb vendors at the farmers' market what grows well in your area. Many will have excellent tips about how to work your soil and what varieties do well where you live. This is a process you'll have to repeat with each move. For example, when I relocated to North Carolina, it was the first time I had a garden with soil that had a lot of clay. Having neighbors who gardened and who had a good relationship with the farmers at the market was tremendously helpful, since the knowledge I had gained by gardening in New York, Vermont, and Switzerland didn't apply under the new conditions I faced.

When planting your herb garden, try to plant from seeds as much as possible. This saves money, of course, and it also teaches you about gardening and what grows well in your area. Don't be concerned with straight-as-an-arrow row planting or pulling every last weed. Gardening is supposed to be a fun stress reliever. Just trust in the process and allow yourself to observe the journey from seed to harvest.

WILDCRAFTING

Wildcrafting simply means gathering plants from the wild—from fields, meadows, mountainsides, natural areas, pastures, or anywhere you can legally pick herbs. If you are not on public lands, request permission from the property owner. Many people skip this step and don't ask—that is a great way to get someone mad at you. Most people, I've discovered, are tickled to let you pick wild plants from their pastures,

IDENTIFYING WILD HERB PLANTS

A good field guide can be your most important tool if you plan to pick herbs in the wild. I recommend the following books:

- *A Field Guide to Medicinal Plants and Herbs of Eastern and Central North America* by Steven Foster, James Duke, and Roger Tory Peterson (A similar version of this Peterson Field Guide covers western medicinal plants and herbs.)
- *Botany in a Day* by Thomas Elpel
- *Field Guide to Medicinal Wild Plants* by Bradford Angier
- *Growing 101 Herbs That Heal: Gardening Techniques, Recipes, and Remedies* by Tammi Hartung
- *Identifying and Harvesting Edible and Medicinal Plants* by Steve Brill

In addition to toting along a good field guide, several other strategies can help you identify plants in the field. Here are some tips:

- Always carry a camera and take pictures of plants you don't recognize so you can look them up later.
- Hire a local guide to lead identification walks. Many botanical societies, gardening clubs, Boy or Girl Scout troops, organic gardening associations, nature preserves, forest preserves, natural food stores, and alternative health clinics can recommend someone. Some localities now have small herb festivals and herb walks. Local publications often feature this information.
- Plant herbs yourself and label them with name stakes. Then you'll be able to identify them when you see them in the wild.

fields, and woods, as long as you are polite and respectful to them and the land. You never know: you may also make a new friend.

I believe wildcrafting has a spiritual aspect. Native Americans and others who practice nature-based religions ask before taking and always give something back to the earth. Traditionally, indigenous people have used tobacco, cornmeal, or another valued commodity as a special offering. We are all indigenous people of the planet, so we should all give back. Think about what you can give back when you take. Planting roots or seeds is a great way to replenish and give back, as is donating to conservation projects.

Whether or not you share my beliefs, you should follow certain rules when wildcrafting, not only for how to pick the herbs but also for respecting nature. Following are the steps I take:

BEFORE GATHERING ANY HERBS, STUDY THE ENVIRONMENT. Never pick herbs in contaminated habitats, such as areas along highways, beside factories, or near any other structure that may have tainted the earth. Do not pick herbs that are growing where you see dead and dying plants, garbage in the undergrowth, oil-slicked puddles, or sewage. Remember that plants store the environment's energy, water, and air. If the area is polluted, then the herb is most likely polluted as well.

Never harvest more than you can use, and never deplete a local plant stand. I often tell my students not to pick more than 10 percent of an existing herbal stand or patch. (However, that percentage can vary depending on the size of the patch.) Other people in the community may also want to harvest the plants. Also consider that animals and insects rely on plants for food, pollination, and other necessities.

DO NOT PICK PROTECTED PLANTS. Find out which plants are protected in your area and use a good field guide to identify them. Just because a plant appears to be plentiful does not mean you can pick it. And a plant that is not protected in one area may be protected in another, so find out which plants are protected wherever you wildcraft. If in doubt, don't harvest the plant. Information about protected plants can be found on state wildlife websites (most will have a link to this information) and the USDA website (plants.usda.gov) under the threatened and endangered listings.

HARVESTING HERBS

Harvest time is best determined by the herb's growth stage rather than by a specific date or month. Most herbs are ready to be harvested just as the flower buds appear. At this stage of growth, the herb's leaves contain the maximum amount of volatile oils, giving the greatest flavor and fragrance to the finished product.

Herbs should be collected in dry weather. If it's been damp all season, let the plants air-dry on a towel before using. Turn them often to help them dry out.

When you want to use fresh herbs, simply pick a few leaves or sprigs here and there as needed throughout the season. If you are harvesting a lot at one time for drying, leave some of the foliage so the plant can continue to grow. Careful pruning ensures new growth.

Harvesting Different Kinds of Plants

Plants are harvested at varying times and with varying methods. Following are some guidelines for harvesting different types of plants according to their seasonal growth cycles.

Annuals

Annuals, such as basil, complete their growth in one season. Trim them during the growing season any time you need a few leaves. Use a sharp knife, scissors, or pruning shears to cut just above a leaf or a pair of leaves, allowing four to six inches of the stem to remain for later growth. (Do not harvest leaves from plants that you are growing for seed. Allow the plants to mature fully before harvesting the seed and the leaves.) In the fall, annuals can be cut back quite severely—if not uprooted and removed from the garden completely—since they will not regenerate or grow back unless reseeded.

When harvesting annuals, take no more than 60 percent of the foliage from most annuals at any one harvest. When harvesting short-lived annuals, such as coriander and dill, cut the whole stalk once and then replant for a new crop.

Perennials

Perennials, such as lavender, die back on their own and produce new growth the next season. Most perennial herbs will be ready to harvest just prior to or during the early part of July, with a second harvest possible in September in most parts of the United States. Only about one-third of the top growth should be removed at a time. In some cases, only the leafy tips should be removed. At the end of the growing season, cut them about halfway down. For the final seasonal harvest of perennials, leave about half the foliage on the plants.

Biennials

Biennials, such as anise and parsley, require two growing seasons to go to seed. They may reseed themselves if they are organic and not genetically modified. Consider them short-term perennials. Leaves may be harvested the first year, but I think it is better to wait until the plant is in its second year. At the end of the growing season, cut biennials about halfway down. When harvesting biennial herbs, pick the leaves as needed the first year, but wait until the seeds set the second year to increase your supply of plants.

Harvesting Different Parts of Plants

In herbalism, all different parts of a plant, such as flowers, leaves, and roots, are used. Not all parts of a plant are harvested at the same time or in the same way. To harvest specific parts of a plant, refer to the following guidelines.

Bark

Bark is harvested in both the spring and fall because that's when the sap of the plant is running. In the spring, the sap runs from the roots upward to the parts of the plant that are above ground. The reverse is true in the fall.

Bark should peel easily from the wood. Never cut through bark in a solid line around the trunk; this will kill the tree. It's best to take bark from wood that has already been felled. Harvest bark from broken branches, twigs, and peeling sections. You can also use bark from branches that have been recently pruned. Do not use bark from rotting or dead branches.

Flowers

Flowers usually contain the best medicine the plant has to offer, so harvest them right after they have fully opened. Do not take broken, bruised, or diseased flowers.

Leaves

Leaves should be gathered in their prime. The optimum time to collect leaves is in clear, dry weather, in the morning after the dew is gone and the sun is still low. Leaves have the most volatile oils at this time. Do not harvest leaves that are contaminated, discolored, or diseased. If you're gathering a flowering plant, harvest just before the plant flowers or immediately after full flowering occurs. (During flowering, the plant is giving most of its energy to make beautiful flowers.)

Roots

Roots should be harvested in the fall when the plants are dormant. At any other time of the growing season, the roots are circulating nutrients and energy to feed the plant's foliage. (To remember this, use the herb gatherer's saying: "Nutrients and healing power fall to the root; in spring, they spring to the plant.") Roots hold the plant's lifeblood and should be collected in a manner that honors this. When digging roots, try to leave some of the root so the plant can continue to grow and produce.

To harvest roots you will need a strong shovel or trowel and a container to put the roots in. I like to use a light canvas bag because the bag's texture removes a substantial amount of surface dirt from the roots. A box or paper bag also works fine. While the roots are still in the bag, remove as much dirt from them as you can, then pour out the excess dirt. Alternatively, wear a pair of canvas gloves and rub the roots with your hands to achieve the same effect. When you get home, use a vegetable brush under running water to wash off as much of the remaining dirt as you can, as quickly as you can, so the root won't absorb water and become soft. Let the root dry completely. Using a fresh, wet root will cause your remedies to spoil, especially if they are oil based. Many roots come out pretty clean, others will be caked with soil, depending on the plant, the water content of the soil, and the type of root.

Seeds

Seeds should be harvested in their prime. This isn't always easy because they tend to fall off or float away in the breeze when they're ready. To harvest seeds, collect the seed heads when they are turning brown by cutting them off the plants. Dry the seeds on a screen or a tray made of very fine wire mesh. Store them in a covered jar or tin in a cool, dark, and dry spot until needed. So that they will germinate when planted in the spring, some herb seeds have to be frozen in advance. Be sure to find out if this is true for the seed you're collecting. Obviously, this is only important if you plan to plant the seed.

PRESERVING HERBS

Preserving fresh herbs guarantees that you'll have a supply to carry you through the season. If you want to store your herbs for more than a few days, you can either dry them or freeze them. Air-drying is the traditional method, oven drying and freezing are quicker, and microwave drying is handy for small batches. Remove all damaged, discolored, or diseased leaves before trying one of the following methods.

Drying

For medicinal uses, dried herbs are usually preferable to fresh ones, because they contain more concentrated amounts of the herb's active ingredients. Dried herbs are easy to store and keep exceedingly well, so you'll always have herbs readily available.

There are many ways to dry herbs, from using elaborate screening trays in a greenhouse to using the oven in your kitchen. The important thing to remember is that no matter how you dry herbs—whether you hang them from the barn rafters or zap them in your microwave—the point is to dry them, not cook them.

Most herbs can be dried, but there are exceptions. Garlic and stinging nettles should always be used fresh or frozen because their active compounds deteriorate when they are dried. Also, when possible, use freshly picked echinacea plants instead of dried.

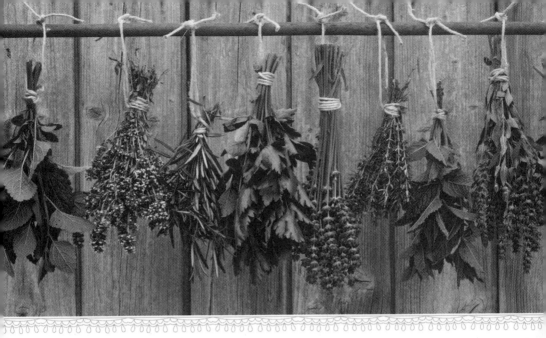

When drying whole branches or stems, strip off the flowers, small leaves, and very small stems. Wash the branches or stems under cool water and gently pat them dry with a dish towel or paper towel. Gather five to eight stems together and tie them into a bundle with twine or kitchen string. Put the bundle in a brown paper bag with the stems extending out of the open end and tie the bag closed around the stems. Hang the bag in a dark, warm place (70 to 80 degrees F). Depending on the temperature and humidity, drying time will take two to four weeks.

Air-Drying

Air-drying is a time-honored technique for preserving herbs. Leafy herbs are usually hung upside down to dry. Gather fresh herbs in a small bunch of three to five stems each for large, leafy herbs, such as sage, or six to eight stems each for smaller herbs, such as thyme.

Secure the stem end of each bundle with a rubber band. To dry seeds, hang the seed heads on their stalks upside down in a paper bag. The seeds will fall into the bag as they dry. Most herbs will dry to the touch in one to three days, depending on the amount of humidity in the air.

Dehydrating

You can use a food dehydrator to dry herbs. I recommend the Nesco American Harvest and Excalibur dehydrators. You can also get good-quality dehydrators from businesses that cater to the raw-food community. Follow the manufacturer's instructions.

Oven Drying

A conventional gas or electric oven, or even a microwave oven (see below), can be used to dry herbs quickly. This must be done carefully, though, because drying herbs too quickly at too high a temperature results in the loss of flavor, oils, and color.

To dry herbs in an electric oven, preheat the oven to 100 degrees F. This may not be possible in modern ovens that do not have warming drawers or a setting as low as 100 degrees. In a gas oven, the heat from the pilot light is ideal for drying herbs; there's no need to turn on the oven. Many modern gas ovens do not have pilot lights, however, so this option may not available to you. Put the leaves and stems on a baking sheet or in a shallow pan and dry them in the oven for three to four hours with the oven door open.

Roots take longer to dry because of their thickness. Roots that can be dried successfully include burdock, comfrey, ginger, ginseng, and sassafras. To dry roots, first scrub them clean with a brush. Slice larger roots in half lengthwise; smaller roots may be left whole. Preheat the oven to 175 degrees F. Put the roots in a shallow pan and dry them in the oven for three to four hours with the oven door cracked.

Microwave Drying

Some herbs with flowers, as well as just the petals alone, maintain extremely good color, form, and flavor when dried in the microwave. Others, though, seem to cook and become crispy but flavorless. Experiment to see which herbs dry best.

In a microwave-safe dish, lay out clean stems or leaves evenly on paper towels. Put another layer of paper towels on top of the herbs. Heat in the microwave on high for one to three minutes, turning the stems or stirring the leaves every thirty seconds. Keep a close eye on the drying herbs and turn off the microwave if you see any signs of smoke or charring. If this happens, try drying a new batch for a shorter period of time. When you determine the right drying time, jot it down for future reference.

I do not advocate the microwave method. I think microwaves disturb the herb's energy, but that's just my opinion. As an herbalist, it's my job to supply options, and some people might find using a microwave convenient. Ultimately, we all have to do whatever works for our lifestyles and families.

Salt Drying

Herbs can also be dried in salt. Salt draws moisture from the herbs and absorbs some of their essential oils. You can use the flavored salt to season your food. To make herbed seasoning salt to sprinkle on foods, wash, dry, and mince the leaves of the herbs you want to use.

To preserve sprigs to crumble into foods, wash and dry sprigs of the herbs you want to use, then remove and discard any thick stems or inedible parts. Salt drying works best with thin-leaved herbs, such as dill, rosemary, savory, tarragon, and thyme. You can also dry thicker herbs in salt—just use fewer leaves and more salt.

To dry herbs with salt, pour kosher salt, sea salt, or another noniodized salt into a container until the salt is one-quarter inch deep. Be sure to use a container that has a tight-fitting lid, such as a canning jar or freezer container. Sprinkle the minced herbs over the salt layer. If you are using sprigs, place them on top of the salt layer. Cover the herbs with another layer of salt, one-quarter inch deep. Continue layering the herbs and salt until you've used up all the herbs. End with a layer of salt. Cover the container and seal tightly.

The herbs will dry in about a week. To make seasoning salt, mix the salt and herbs together well, then pour the mixture into a small, airtight container to keep on your kitchen counter or table. To use the dried sprigs, simply pull out individual sprigs, brush off the salt, and crumble the herbs into food.

Tray Drying

Tray drying is usually used for short-stemmed herbs, such as thyme, or for individual leaves, such as basil. You can use an old window screen or make your own small drying tray with a 2 x 2-inch piece of lumber and a cloth or screen. Wash and dry the herbs, then lay them out on the drying tray. Keep the tray in a warm, dark place until the herbs are dry. Leaves will require a couple of days to a week to dry; flowers, about two weeks; and thinly sliced roots, up to a month. The time it takes for an herb to dry thoroughly will depend on the type of herb, the humidity, and the temperature.

Freezing

Freezing is a quick and easy way to preserve many herbs. It's especially good for herbs that tend to lose their flavor when dried, such as basil, chives, French tarragon, lovage, and parsley. When the frozen herbs are thawed, however, they are limp and not especially attractive, so they're best used in teas, tinctures, and syrups.

To prepare leaves for freezing, chop them and put them in plastic containers or bags. Another method is to purée herbs in a blender with a little water or olive oil and freeze the purée in ice-cube trays. When the easy-to-use cubes are ready, remove them from the trays and store them in plastic containers or bags in the freezer. Label all frozen herbs with their date of storage and use them within six months.

Making Candy

American colonists couldn't run to the store to buy candy when they had a sweet tooth, so they made their own sweet treats out of herbs. They candied young angelica stems and ginger, preserving the herb and bringing out its flavor with a crystal-sugar shell. Although their sweets may not replace modern candies, they are wonderful as dessert garnishes or edible decorations on cakes and pastries.

Cookbooks from the 1700s recommended the following process for candied angelica: Cook young angelica stems in boiling water until tender. Peel off and discard the fibrous strings. Return the stems to simmering water and cook until they turn very green. Remove the stems from the water and let them dry. Transfer the dried, cooked stems to a bowl or tray. Cover the stems with an equal amount of superfine granulated white sugar (one pound of sugar per one pound of stems). Let stand for two days. Put the mixture in a large saucepan and boil until the sugar melts into clear syrup. Drain off the syrup. Cover with an equal amount of sugar (again, one pound of sugar per one pound of stems). Remove the stems from the sugar and put them on plates to dry in a warm place. Store in an airtight container.

Making Syrup

Sugar syrups flavored with herbs can add taste to cold drinks and baked foods. Syrups can also be used medicinally. To make herb-flavored sugar syrup, put 2 parts water and 1 part sugar in a saucepan and bring to a simmer. Add a handful of fresh herbs, stems and all, to the simmering syrup. Cook until the herbs lose their color and the syrup is aromatic, 15 to 30 minutes. Use the syrup immediately. Alternatively, let the syrup cool and store it in covered jars in the refrigerator.

STORING HERBS

Store dried herbs in sterilized, dark glass containers with airtight lids. Label the container with the name of the herb, including its Latin genus and species name, and the date. (Labeling is very important. Many dried herbs look and smell alike, making it easy to use the wrong herb, which could be dangerous.) Store dried herbs at room temperature in a cool, dry place away from sunlight, moisture, children, and pets.

Another method is to put herbs in labeled freezer bags and keep them in the freezer for up to six months. You can also store herbs

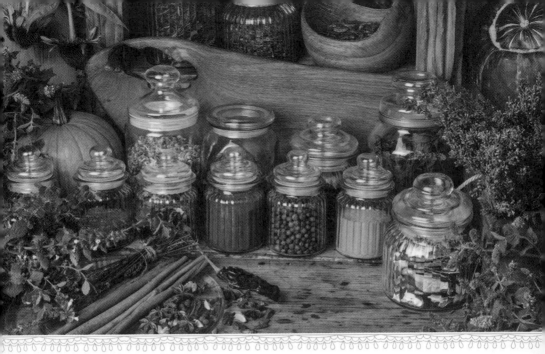

in brown paper bags, which must be kept dry and away from light to prevent bleaching. To keep bugs away, put the paper bags inside plastic containers.

Because moisture can cause herbs to mold, make sure herbs are completely dry before they are stored. If you open a container of stored herbs and find mold, discard the herbs. Do not use moldy herbs.

Dried herbs, except for a few types of roots, have a relatively short life span. Dried flowers, leaves, roots, and other herb parts keep for about one year when stored at or just below room temperature.

In traditional Chinese medicine, practitioners use very old roots; however, in Western herbalism, herbs generally are not considered to have a long shelf life. If you've dried more herbs than you're going to use, consider freezing them. Wrap them in freezer paper and put the wrapped packet in a ziplock bag or a plastic freezer container.

EQUIPMENT

Once you have the herbs, gather together the equipment you'll need to make remedies. This includes saucepans and pots of various sizes, including a six-quart saucepan and a stockpot. Stainless steel, copper, or enamel-coated pans are best. Do not use aluminum, Teflon-coated, or other types of coated cookware.

Because herbal medicines are often served as teas, you will also need high-quality china teapots that can withstand boiling water and a lot of use. Use a cup strainer when pouring the tea.

Following is a list of additional equipment you might need. None of this has to be fancy. You probably have most of these items in your kitchen already:

- baking sheets, two uncoated, heavy gauge (adjust baking time for insulated sheets)
- bottles and jars, glass (reuse baby-food, canning, and small condiment jars or buy new jars for this purpose)
- canning jars and lids
- cheesecloth or muslin
- double boiler
- droppers or pipettes
- French press coffeepot (can be used instead of a teapot or to strain tinctures)
- measuring cups, glass
- measuring spoons, stainless steel
- metal funnels, two or three in different sizes
- muslin bags, 8- and 12-inch
- orifice reducers (to adjust the size of bottle openings)
- salve pots, 2- to 4-ounce glass, and lids
- screening material or window screens for drying herbs
- spray bottles
- strainers, all types, including tea strainers

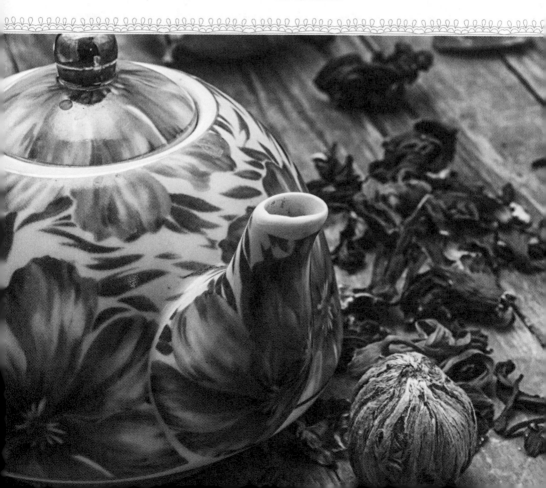

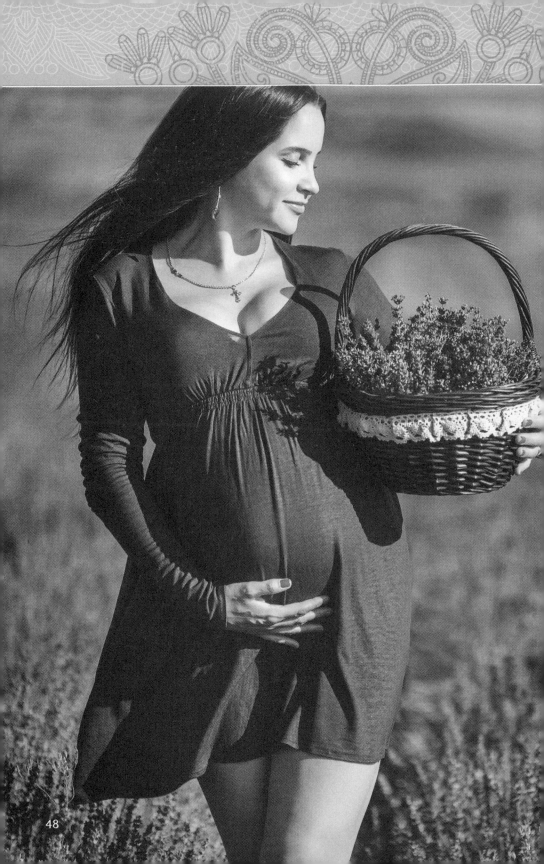

Herbs for Pregnancy, Labor, and Breastfeeding

This section includes herbs that are commonly used during pregnancy, labor, or the postpartum period, when a main concern is breastfeeding. As indicated, some herbs should not be used during pregnancy or when breastfeeding but are helpful during labor. Others can be used during the postpartum period but should not be used before the birth.

In addition, this chapter includes a list of herbs that should not be used at any time unless you're under the direction of a competent health care provider (see page 68). Also included is a short list of culinary herbs that can be used in food preparation but should not be consumed in large amounts (see page 75).

The following lists contain scientific terms that may be unfamiliar. For example, "abortifacient" is a word used to refer to herbs that can cause contractions and abortions. The Glossary (page 171) supplies definitions for many of the terms used in this chapter. In addition, note that this chapter applies only to herbs and not to essential oils, which are listed in chapter 2, "Essential Oils for Pregnancy, Labor, and the Postpartum Period," pages 17 to 27.

HERB DESCRIPTIONS AND SAFETY PROFILES

Alfalfa (Medicago sativa)

Alfalfa is one of the most nutritious herbs. People of all ages, from children to seniors, can benefit from using it. During pregnancy and the postpartum period, alfalfa can provide nourishment, discourage fatigue, and increase a nursing mother's milk supply. In general, it's good for overall health, is a gentle diuretic, and stimulates the appetite. Alfalfa also may be beneficial for reducing cholesterol.

A nutritional superstar, alfalfa is up to 50 percent protein and quite rich in calcium; in fact, the ashes of its leaves are almost 99 percent pure calcium. Other featured minerals include copper, iron, magnesium, phosphorus, potassium, and zinc. A powerhouse when it comes to vitamin K, alfalfa also contains vitamins A, B_1, B_6, B_{12}, C, D, and E; biotin; folic acid; niacin; and pantothenic acid. In addition, alfalfa provides plentiful amino acids, beta-carotene, chlorophyll, flavonoids, saponins, and sterols.

CONTRAINDICATIONS: None known.

Aloe vera (Aloe vera)

When aloe vera gel is taken fresh from the plant's leaves and applied topically, it has superior wound-healing abilities. Commercially sold gels can also be helpful but contain preservatives, which can cause stinging. In addition, whatever the source, the gel can cause some yellow staining, which is not harmful and washes off easily with soap and water. Because aloe vera gel has a high water content, users must allow the skin to dry after application.

The gel contains powerful plant sterols, which have an anti-inflammatory effect like steroid drugs but don't inhibit healing like drugs. That's why it's so effective in treating dry skin. Allantoin, a substance in aloe vera, promotes skin growth. In addition, it has been shown that aloe vera increases collagen content in skin. Studies demonstrated that collagen increased 93 percent with topical aloe vera treatment, compared to controls.

Aloe vera leaves, which are sold in dried form, act as a strong laxative. They should not be taken internally.

CONTRAINDICATIONS: Topical use of aloe vera gel during pregnancy has no known side effects. Taking it internally is not considered safe during pregnancy or when breastfeeding.

Angelica (Angelica archangelica)

When given in high doses, angelica is a uterine stimulant. It may be used after a birth to successfully deliver the placenta, even if the placenta is fully adhered. Angelica (*Angelica archangelica*) should not be confused with dong quai (*Angelica sinensis*), which can exacerbate bleeding. As a culinary herb, angelica is quite safe.

Anise, aniseeds *(Pimpinella anisum)*

Although safe when used as a culinary herb, high doses of anise or aniseeds can act as a uterine stimulant, warranting some caution during pregnancy. In general, anise and aniseeds are used to ease colic, constipation, gas, indigestion, and spasmodic intestinal pain.

Arnica *(Arnica montana)*

Made from arnica flowers, arnica creams, gels, and sprays can be purchased or made at home. Arnica-infused oils are very effective in treating bruises. Any of these remedies can be used topically during pregnancy. Note, however, that arnica-infused oil should not be used on broken skin. Arnica should not be taken internally unless in a homeopathic remedy.

NOTE: Topical remedies made from arnica the herb should not be confused with arnica essential oil (page 23), which is not safe to use during pregnancy.

Basil *(Ocimum basilicum)*

As a culinary herb, basil is found in many Mediterranean dishes and considered quite safe. In medicinal doses, this herb is often contraindicated during pregnancy but can be useful after the baby's birth when the placenta is being delivered. In general, basil can be beneficial for treating menstrual issues and relieving insomnia and stress.

Beth root *(Trillium erectum)*

A uterine stimulant, Beth root, which is also called trillium, is traditionally used at the onset of labor and can cause strong uterine contractions. In fact, the herb has long been used for this purpose in the United States, first by indigenous people and then by European settlers. In addition, Beth root is used prior to labor to smooth the progress of contractions and make the delivery easier. Used after delivery, Beth root can decrease the incidence and severity of postpartum hemorrhage.

Bitter melon *(Momordica charantia)*

An herb that can be beneficial in treating gestational diabetes, bitter melon should be used during pregnancy only with professional guidance. This is the case because overuse can cause uterine contractions.

CONTRAINDICATIONS: When too much is used during early pregnancy, bitter melon has been linked to stinging contractions. As the term suggests, these contractions cause a stinging feeling in the abdomen.

Black cohosh *(Cimicifuga racemosa)*

Because black cohosh can cause premature contractions, it should be used during pregnancy only with professional guidance. Black cohosh relieves muscle pain, which is one reason it works so well with blue cohosh (see opposite page), the uterine stimulant. Together, the combo is considered the best to have on hand for births. Black cohosh is not only excellent as a liniment for back labor, but it's also used to relieve pain and cramping in the womb.

After more than forty years of observed use in Germany, black cohosh has shown no serious adverse effects, contraindications, or drug interactions. Studies have concluded that the herb does not cause defects or mutations. In addition, it's not a carcinogen.

Grown in the United States and Canada, black cohosh is rich in volatile oils, isoflavones, and other beneficial components. It is an alterative, antispasmodic, emmenagogic, hypotensive, and nervine.

CONTRAINDICATIONS: Black cohosh should not be used during early pregnancy because it can stimulate uterine contractions.

Black haw *(Viburnum prunifolium)*

Black haw has a long history of being used for clinical ripening, which refers to a softening of the cervix that must occur so that dilation can begin. Black haw is also used to soothe afterpains, which the mother experiences after the baby is born.

CONTRAINDICATIONS: Black haw should be used during pregnancy only with professional guidance. In addition, remedies made with black haw should not be used by anyone who is allergic to aspirin.

Black pepper *(Piper nigrum)*

Generally considered safe since it is a commonly used seasoning, black pepper may be recommended by herbalists to stimulate digestion, improve blood circulation, and warm the body.

Black tea *(Camellia sinensis)*

Drinking black tea can be beneficial for people who experience fatigue and headaches, although the limit should be two cups per day. More than that can cause heart palpitations and an increased heart rate. In addition, black tea is used in topical applications and is a good choice for treating swelling and inflamed tissues.

CONTRAINDICATIONS: No more than two cups of black tea should be consumed per day.

Black walnut (Juglans nigra)

Black walnut is used to treat pain. In addition, because it's an antiviral, it can be used to help prevent a herpes outbreak.

CONTRAINDICATIONS: Black walnut should not be taken internally during pregnancy or when nursing.

Blackberry leaves (Rubus fruticosus)

Blackberry leaves are an excellent and quick-acting herbal remedy for diarrhea. As an astringent, this herb is used topically to treat varicose veins and is particularly effective when used in baths, compresses, and washes.

CONTRAINDICATIONS: None known.

Blessed thistle (Cnicus benedictus)

Safe to use during the postpartum period, blessed thistle can increase a nursing mother's milk supply. It is also helpful for treating postpartum headaches.

CONTRAINDICATIONS: Blessed thistle should not be used during pregnancy. In addition, this herb should not be used by anyone who is allergic to plants in the Asteraceae family.

Blue cohosh (Caulophyllum thalictroides)

Blue cohosh is an antispasmodic and can be used at any time during pregnancy if there is a threat of miscarriage. Also because of its antispasmodic action, blue cohosh will ease false labor pains during pregnancy. Safe to use during childbirth, the herb can help induce labor. In addition, during labor, the use of blue cohosh just previous to birth will ease delivery. When given after birth, blue cohosh can lessen bleeding and help deliver a retained placenta because it makes the uterus contract without closing the cervix. Grown in the United States and Canada, blue cohosh is an emmenagogue and diuretic.

CONTRAINDICATIONS: Blue cohosh should be used during pregnancy only with professional guidance because it stimulates uterine contractions. It should not be used during early pregnancy. There is in vitro evidence that blue cohosh may cross the placental membrane, disturb growth and development, and have potentially toxic effects on the embryo.

Borage *(Borago officinalis)*

A source of calcium and potassium, borage is a culinary herb and generally considered safe. Used to treat anxiety and depression, borage is also a tonic for the adrenals. Borage should not be confused with borage seed oil, which is used differently.

Burdock root *(Arctium lappa)*

Traditionally used as a vegetable in Asian dishes, burdock root is generally considered safe for consumption as a food, except during pregnancy. However, it can be used topically during pregnancy and may be added to sitz baths and washes to soothe eczema or PUPPP (see page 123).

Calendula flowers *(Calendula officinalis)*

Used to make infused oil, compresses, and sitz baths, calendula can be very soothing. Because it is an anti-inflammatory, astringent, and vulnerary, it softens skin, reduces inflammation, and promotes wound healing. In addition, it is antimicrobial.

CONTRAINDICATIONS: Although calendula is extremely safe for topical use, it should not be taken orally during pregnancy. In addition, it should not be used by anyone who is allergic to plants in the Asteraceae and Compositae families.

Canada fleabane or Canadian horseweed *(Conyza canadensis, formerly Erigeron canadensis)*

Canadian fleabane is traditionally used to stem postpartum bleeding.

Caraway seeds *(Carum carvi)*

Considered quite safe as a culinary herb, caraway seeds can be a uterine stimulant when used in higher doses. As a galactagogue, it's beneficial for promoting breast-milk production.

CONTRAINDICATIONS: Caraway seeds should not be used during early pregnancy because they can cause the uterus to relax. In addition, they should not be used by anyone who is allergic to caraway oil.

Cardamom *(Elettaria cardamomum)*

A culinary herb that is generally considered safe, cardamom is commonly used to treat digestion problems, including constipation, gas, heartburn, intestinal spasms, and irritable bowel syndrome. It can also stimulate appetite and relieve gallbladder and liver complaints. In general, cardamom is beneficial for treating bronchitis, the common cold, cough, sore mouth, and sore throat, and it can help ward off infection.

Catnip *(Nepeta cataria)*

Catnip shares many of the same properties as German and Roman chamomile (see below) and can be used instead of or in combination with chamomile.

CONTRAINDICATIONS: Catnip can cause uterine contractions during early pregnancy.

Chamomile, German *(Matricaria chamomilla)*

German chamomile is known for reducing inflammation. It can be made into an infused oil, a salve, or a bath tea. In general, German and Roman chamomile can be used interchangeably. Although they belong to different species, they are often used to treat similar health problems.

CONTRAINDICATIONS: Overall, German chamomile is reputed to be very safe. However, it can cause problems for people who use blood-thinning medications or are allergic to ragweed.

Chamomile, Roman *(Anthemis nobilis)*

A well-documented anti-inflammatory herb, chamomile is effective in reducing intestinal, mouth and throat, and skin inflammation. In addition, it is a gentle herb that eases aches, cramps, low back pain, and spasms. During the postpartum period, it promotes breast-milk production, is calming for the mother, and may help prevent or relieve colic in the baby. In general, Roman and German chamomile (see above) can be used interchangeably. Although they belong to different species, they are often used to treat similar health problems.

CONTRAINDICATIONS: Roman chamomile is generally considered safe but should not be used by people who are allergic to ragweed or other plants in the Asteraceae family.

Chaparral *(Larrea tridentate)*

Chaparral is used topically for a variety of issues, especially to decrease inflammation and pain and to promote healing of minor wounds. A compress soaked in infused oil or herb tea can be applied several times a day for these concerns, and heat can be added if it's helpful. As a well-known herbal antibiotic, powdered chaparral can be applied directly to minor wounds after they have been properly cleansed. Chaparral can also be used in a sitz bath.

CONTRAINDICATIONS: Chaparral should not be taken internally. Considered unsafe for use by nursing mothers, it can potentially cause serious liver and kidney problems.

Chickweed *(Stellaria media)*

A favorite during pregnancy, chickweed is soothing when used topically as a compress, an infused oil, or a poultice or when added to a sitz bath. As an emollient and vulnerary, it is a common topical remedy for itching and irritation as well as cuts and wounds. Rich in vitamin C and bioflavonoids, it can help reduce scarring. When the baby arrives, chickweed is a good choice for infant skin care. In addition, chickweed can be eaten as a nutritious salad herb.

CONTRAINDICATIONS: None known.

Cinnamon *(Cinnamomum zeylanicum)*

Cinnamon is often used to aid digestion and relieve stomach cramps and pain. Effective for maintaining a healthy balance of blood sugar, cinnamon may help control diabetes. More studies are being done on this.

CONTRAINDICATIONS: Cinnamon is a culinary herb and generally considered safe when used in small amounts; however, it should not be used in large quantities. Doses of one teaspoon or more may have narcotic effects, potentially causing convulsions, delirium, hallucinations, and even death in adults.

Cleavers *(Galium aparine)*

Generally considered safe, cleavers can lower blood pressure and is a slight diuretic. Used topically, it provides relief for skin that is irritated by incontinence, eczema, or sores.

CONTRAINDICATIONS: None known.

Clove *(Syzygium aromaticum)*

As a culinary herb, clove is generally considered safe. In an herbal tea, it is beneficial for treating nausea and eliminating excess gas in the stomach and intestines, which can be welcome during pregnancy and the postpartum period. Gas can be especially problematic after a C-section. Clove is also beneficial for treating pain.

Comfrey *(Symphytum officinale)*

As an anti-inflammatory, comfrey is used topically to treat a number of injuries. In a compress or poultice, it is especially helpful for treating external ulcers, fractures, and wounds. In fact, comfrey can speed wound healing and deter the development of scar tissue. Care should be taken with very deep wounds, however, because applying comfrey can cause tissue to form over the wound before it has healed deeper down, potentially leading to an abscess. In addition, comfrey may decrease bruising.

CONTRAINDICATIONS: Although topical use is generally considered safe, comfrey should not be taken internally during pregnancy, in part because it contains alkaloids that have abortifacient effects. In general, I rarely suggest that comfrey be taken internally because there is some controversy about its safety.

Coriander (Coriandrum sativum)

Coriander is a general remedy for anxiety, insomnia, nervous tension, and stress. During late pregnancy, it is used for overall digestive support and to relieve upset stomach. After a C-section, coriander eases the gas pains associated with surgery.

CONTRAINDICATIONS: Coriander is generally considered to be safe, although some sources indicate that medicinal doses should not be used during pregnancy.

Corn silk (Zea mays)

Corn silk has traditionally been used for urinary disorders and is known for effectively treating inflammation in the urinary system and kidneys. As a gentle diuretic, it helps the body flush out contaminants by increasing urination.

CONTRAINDICATIONS: None known.

Cottonwood bark (Gossypium hirsutum)

A good herb for treating postpartum pain, cottonwood bark is traditionally used to treat gastrointestinal issues, such as diarrhea and nausea. It is also used to relieve fever, headache, hemorrhage, and pain. In addition, it's useful for managing menstrual issues.

CONTRAINDICATIONS: Cottonwood bark can cause strong uterine contractions and should not be used during pregnancy.

Couch grass (Agropyron repens)

Couch grass is a safe diuretic. In addition, it is a demulcent that soothes irritation and inflammation.

CONTRAINDICATIONS: None known.

Cramp bark (Viburnum opulus)

As the name suggests, cramp bark is beneficial for easing both muscular cramps and the pain associated with cramping and spasms. It also relaxes the uterus and other smooth muscles, such as blood vessels and bronchial mucous membranes.

CONTRAINDICATIONS: Cramp bark should be used during pregnancy only with professional guidance. People who use blood-thinning medications should not use cramp bark. In addition, its berries are toxic and should not be used.

Dandelion *(Taraxacum officinale)*

As a culinary herb and food, dandelion is generally considered safe. Dried leaves and roots are typically infused as a tea, and fresh leaves are added to salads or steamed. Dandelion leaves are rich in vitamins, specifically vitamins A, C, and K, and are good sources of calcium, iron, manganese, and potassium. In general, dandelion promotes good digestion and bile production.

CONTRAINDICATIONS: Dandelion is a potent diuretic, and this fact should be considered before use.

Devil's claw *(Harpagophytum procumbens)*

Although it's not safe to use during pregnancy, devil's claw is a good choice for treating nerve pain during labor and incontinence problems during the postpartum period. In general, the herb is used topically to relieve sore muscles and joints.

CONTRAINDICATIONS: Devil's claw is a uterine stimulant and should not be used during pregnancy.

Dill *(Anethum graveolens)*

Dill is a common culinary herb that adds flavor to savory dishes. It is generally considered safe, although it can act as a uterine stimulant. It is frequently included in herbal remedies for breastfeeding.

Echinacea root *(Echinacea purpurea)*

Echinacea is primarily valued for the role it plays in supporting the immune system. In addition, it's an effective anti-inflammatory.

CONTRAINDICATIONS: Overall, echinacea is considered very safe, but it should not be used by anyone who is allergic to ragweed.

Fennel *(Foeniculum vulgare)*

Fennel is an exceptional stomach and intestinal remedy. It not only stimulates the appetite and digestion but also relieves flatulence. During the postpartum period, fennel is used to promote breast-milk production. This herb has a sweet, mellow flavor.

CONTRAINDICATIONS: Although considered safe as a culinary herb, in high doses fennel can be a uterine stimulant. It should not be used by anyone who is allergic to celery.

Fenugreek (Trigonella foenum-graecum)

Using fenugreek as a culinary herb is quite safe during pregnancy, and it's a beneficial source of soluble fiber. During the postpartum period, fenugreek greatly increases breast-milk production. In general, fenugreek tea aids digestion and eases constipation. In traditional herbal medicine, fenugreek seeds have been used to decrease cholesterol and blood sugar levels.

CONTRAINDICATIONS: Although fenugreek is generally considered safe as a culinary herb, medicinal doses should be used only with professional guidance during pregnancy.

Feverfew flowers (Tanacetum parthenium)

As a uterine stimulant, feverfew has the potential to cause premature contractions. However, it is useful for delivering a delayed placenta.

CONTRAINDICATIONS: Feverfew should not be used during pregnancy.

Garlic (Allium sativum)

High doses of garlic can cause heartburn and affect the flavor of breast milk. Moderate culinary use is typically safe but should be avoided during bouts of heartburn.

CONTRAINDICATIONS: None known.

German chamomile (SEE CHAMOMILE, GERMAN, PAGE 55)

Ginger (Zingiber officinale)

Perhaps best known for its effectiveness in relieving nausea, ginger can be essential during pregnancy and also helpful for motion sickness and chemotherapy nausea. In addition, ginger has a long tradition of being used for osteoarthritis.

CONTRAINDICATIONS: Ginger is generally safe unless it's used excessively.

Ginkgo (Ginkgo biloba)

Ginkgo is beneficial for treating carpal tunnel syndrome, but it should be used only after pregnancy. This is because it may have antiplatelet properties that could prolong bleeding after delivery.

CONTRAINDICATIONS: Ginkgo should be used with caution during pregnancy, particularly near the due date or any time that bleeding occurs.

Gotu kola *(Centella asiatica)*

As a potential emmenagogue, gotu kola should be used carefully and only occasionally during pregnancy. Several scientific studies have documented gotu kola's effectiveness in healing wounds, and the herb is known to promote collagen production, which also aids healing. In addition, gotu kola is a good choice for reducing swelling and increasing circulation.

CONTRAINDICATIONS: Gotu kola should not be used regularly during pregnancy.

Gurmar *(Gymnema sylvestre)*

Gurmar is a commonly used herb in India and has been studied extensively since the 1920s. It may increase the body's production of insulin and encourage the pancreas to develop more beta cells (the source of insulin), making it useful in treating gestational diabetes.

Hibiscus flowers *(Hibiscus sabdariffa)*

Rich in antioxidants, flavonoids, and other nutrients, hibiscus flowers offer cardiac health benefits and are considered helpful for decreasing blood pressure. In fact, a 2004 study published in *Phytomedicine* showed that a daily cup of hibiscus tea is as effective in decreasing blood pressure as the drug captopril. Also good for the nervous system, hibiscus is a favorite remedy for anxiety and stress.

Hops *(Humulus lupulus)*

Hops are used to ease anxiety, insomnia, restlessness, and stress; however, they should not be used during early pregnancy.

CONTRAINDICATIONS: None known after the first trimester.

Horse chestnut *(Aesculus hippocastanum)*

Horse chestnut contains a compound called aescin that acts as an anti-inflammatory and relieves swollen ankles during pregnancy; the same compound makes horse chestnut a good choice for relieving edema (swelling with fluid) following trauma. It also is an astringent that effectively heals tears, making it useful in a postpartum compress or sitz bath. In general, this herb is known for toning and protecting blood vessels. The bark, leaves, and green fruit can all be used in herbal remedies. Because horse chestnut contains resin, I recommend using it in an alcohol-based tincture so that the resin can't be felt. Simply add 2 teaspoons of tincture to 2 to 3 cups of warm water.

Horsetail (Equisetum arvense)

Beneficial for healing and soothing tissues, horsetail is also reputed to decrease the amount of bacteria in the urinary tract.

CONTRAINDICATIONS: None known.

Lady's mantle (Alchemilla vulgaris; Alchemilla xanthochlora)

Lady's mantle gained popularity in the Middle Ages and has been used to treat women ever since; in fact, it is standard in many midwives' herbal materia medicas. As a uterine stimulant, this herb is traditionally used during labor. In particular, the tincture can encourage contractions.

Lavender (Lavendula officinalis)

Lavender is well known for its pain-relieving properties and for keeping infection at bay. Also effective for relieving stress and relaxing tense muscles, it's a good relaxation aid during late pregnancy. Considered safe as a culinary herb and for topical use, lavender can be a uterine stimulant in high doses.

Lemon balm (Melissa officinalis)

Lemon balm has long been used to relieve anxiety. Studies have shown it to be calming, which makes it a useful tool for reducing stress and improving mood and mental alertness. In general, this herb is rich in antioxidants.

CONTRAINDICATIONS: None known.

Licorice (Glycyrrhiza glabra)

Licorice root is one of the most widely used herbs in the world. Considered safe in moderation, licorice is a helpful additive in postpartum teas.

CONTRAINDICATIONS: Although it's considered safe as a culinary herb, licorice can cause water retention in some individuals. People who retain water or have high blood pressure should avoid licorice.

Marshmallow root (Althaea officinalis)

Marshmallow root, including the roots and the flowers, contains large amounts of mucilage, which soothes and softens tissues and promotes healing.

Milky oats (SEE OATS, BELOW)

Motherwort *(Leonurus cardiaca)*

I can think of no better herb to use during labor and the postpartum period than this one; in fact, the Latin name for motherwort means "lion heart." Although it is not typically used during pregnancy before labor begins, motherwort can ease early labor pains if they are premature. During labor, motherwort can alleviate the anxiety, insomnia, restlessness, and tension that some women experience. After childbirth, it is given to help the uterus relax and return to normal size. In general, motherwort is an excellent tonic for both the uterus and the heart, tonifying the former and reducing palpitations in the latter. Grown in the United States, Canada, and Europe, motherwort is classified as an antispasmodic, emmenagogue, and nervine. It can be quite bitter and is often preferred in tincture form.

CONTRAINDICATIONS: A potential uterine stimulant in high doses, motherwort is generally not used before labor. Anyone who has a clotting disorder should not use motherwort.

Nettles *(Urtica dioica)*

Nettles have traditionally been used to strengthen and support the whole body, and they're wonderful to use during pregnancy and when nursing. They contain calcium, iron, magnesium, potassium, and vitamins A, B, and C. This herb is also rich in chlorophyll and is a high-quality source of beta-carotene, tannins, and other beneficial nutrients. When I recommend an herbal for nutritional value, I always suggest nettles and pair them with raspberry leaves.

CONTRAINDICATIONS: People who retain fluid as a result of decreased renal and cardiac function should not use nettles. In addition, nettles have been shown to enhance the effect of the drug diclofenac; anyone using this drug should seek the advice of a health provider before using nettles. Nettles are contraindicated in cases of fluid retention from decreased renal function and decreased cardiac function.

Oats; Milky Oats *(Avena sativa)*

Gentle and nutritious, oats and milky oats are beneficial for soothing the nervous system, decreasing anxiety and stress, and increasing the breast-milk supply. Oats are a traditional choice for treating irritated skin, including eczema, rashes, and PUPPP (see page 123).

CONTRAINDICATIONS: None known.

Parsley *(Petroselinum crispum)*

Safe for normal culinary use, parsley should be used with care during pregnancy because it is a well-known uterine stimulant and can pose a danger to the fetus in higher doses. Safe for topical application, parsley dilates veins and facilitates blood flow, making it a good choice when treating hemorrhoids and varicose veins.

CONTRAINDICATIONS: Parsley should not used when breastfeeding because it can stop the production of breast milk.

Passionflower *(Passiflora incarnata)*

Overall, this herb is safe when used in moderation. It is particularly beneficial for treating anxiety, insomnia, and stress.

CONTRAINDICATIONS: Because passionflower can be a uterine stimulant when taken in high doses, it should be used during pregnancy only with professional guidance.

Pau d'arco *(Tabebuia avellanedae)*

Pau d'arco is a great antifungal and an excellent remedy to use when treating candida overgrowth.

CONTRAINDICATIONS: Pau d'arco should not be taken internally during pregnancy.

Peach leaves *(Prunus persica)*

Peach leaves, which are typically infused as a tea, are known for their effectiveness in treating nausea and vomiting.

CONTRAINDICATIONS: Peach leaves should not be used by anyone who is allergic to peaches.

Peppermint leaves *(Mentha piperita)*

Peppermint is very useful for easing the discomforts of morning sickness, including nausea and upset stomach.

CONTRAINDICATIONS: Peppermint tea can aggravate gastroesophageal reflux disease (GERD) and may promote the flow of bile from the gallbladder and potentially exacerbate gallstone symptoms.

Plantain *(Plantago major; Plantago officinalis)*

Considered a very safe herb, plantain has anti-inflammatory, antimicrobial, astringent, demulcent, and vulnerary properties. Used topically as a compress, an infused oil, or a poultice or in a sitz bath, it is very beneficial for inflamed tissues, such as hemorrhoids and varicose veins.

Raspberry leaves *(Rubus idaeus)*

Raspberry leaves are among the most used and loved herbs for treating women during pregnancy and have been for hundreds of years of documented use. This herb is nourishing, has a soothing effect on the nervous system, and tones the uterus. Although raspberry leaves can be a uterine stimulant, many women use the leaves throughout their pregnancy with no issues, typically in pregnancy tea blends. During labor, this herb supports contractions and checks hemorrhage. In addition, it can be helpful in delivering the placenta.

In general, raspberry leaves are rich in vitamin C and folate as well as calcium, iron, and zinc. Using both the leaves and berries can help prevent anemia. Raspberry leaves also effectively treat bleeding gums, leg cramps, mouth ulcers, and upset stomach. As a gargle, this herb soothes sore throats. As an astringent, it is a helpful aid for diarrhea.

CONTRAINDICATIONS: Raspberry leaves have no known contraindications. Yet some members of the midwifery and medical communities say it shouldn't be used during early pregnancy or by women with a history of miscarriage. This has been neither proved to be true or untrue. However, to be on the safe side, I suggest that women who are at risk for miscarriage wait until the second trimester to drink raspberry leaf tea.

Red clover *(Trifolium pratense)*

Although it should not be used during pregnancy, red clover contains bioflavonoids and isoflavones and is overall a highly nutritious herb. Considered a gentle blood fortifier, red clover can be very beneficial in aiding conception.

CONTRAINDICATIONS: Red clover should not to be used during pregnancy.

Reishi mushroom *(Ganoderma lucidum)*

Reishi mushrooms have wonderful healing properties that are still being discovered. They can be used to treat herpes symptoms as well as protect against radiation damage.

CONTRAINDICATIONS: Because reishi mushrooms can lower blood pressure and potentially cause clotting problems, this herb should be used with advisement.

Roman chamomile (SEE CHAMOMILE, ROMAN, PAGE 55)

Rooibos *(Aspalathus linearis)*

Generally considered safe, rooibos (pronounced roy-biss) is a wonderful, relaxing, and very nutritious tea. Traditionally it has been used for aiding digestion and relieving nervous tension, stress, and skin issues. Now more common in the United States, rooibos can be found in most natural food stores. I suggest trying unflavored varieties with no added milk or sweetener because the tea is naturally mellow and sweet.

Rose hips *(Rosa canina)*

This is one of my favorite herbs. Rose hips taste great and are a nutritional powerhouse, featuring vitamins C, E, and K and calcium, magnesium, and manganese. Rose hips also contain beta-carotene, flavonoids, lycopene, omega-3 and omega-6 fatty acids, and pectin. In addition, this herb is a good source of dietary fiber, making it an effective, gentle laxative that can assist with constipation.

CONTRAINDICATIONS: None known with proper dosage, which is three to four cups of tea per day, using 1 cup of water to 1 teaspoon of dried herb or 2 teaspoons of fresh herb.

Shepherd's purse *(Capsella bursa-pastoris)*

Shepherd's purse has long been the top recommendation for stemming hemorrhage and excessive bleeding. This makes it a standard for postpartum care, although it should not be used until after the placenta has been delivered. In fact, in the United States, shepherd's purse has been used following expulsion of the placenta since the time of the Pilgrims. It's effective because, as a styptic herb, it constricts blood vessels and tissue, lowering blood pressure and contracting the uterus. It is also an astringent, anti-inflammatory, and diuretic. Found in many parts of the world, including Europe, North America, and Asia, shepherd's purse leaves are quite nutritious, providing protein, vitamins C and K, calcium, iron, and sodium.

CONTRAINDICATIONS: Although safe for topical use, shepherd's purse should not be taken internally during pregnancy. However, it can be taken internally during the postpartum period after the placenta has been delivered and when used as directed.

Skullcap *(Scutellaria lateriflora)*

For general use, skullcap is helpful in relieving muscle spasms and pain as well as insomnia, nightmares, and stress.

CONTRAINDICATIONS: Skullcap should be used in limited amounts during pregnancy and only with professional guidance.

Slippery elm *(Ulmus rubra)*

Slippery elm bark is commonly used to make lozenges, and these can be found at most natural food stores. Given slippery elm's emollient property, the lozenges lubricate and coat the esophagus.

CONTRAINDICATIONS: Slippery elm can potentially cause uterine contractions and should be used during pregnancy only with professional guidance.

Spearmint leaves *(Mentha spicata)*

Spearmint is a favorite during pregnancy because it relieves nausea and alleviates morning sickness. A gentler alternative to peppermint, spearmint has traditionally been used for indigestion, nausea, and gas. Spearmint can also be used to decrease muscle spasms in the stomach. High in vitamins A and C, this mint has a good flavor, which can be used to mask the earthy taste of some herbal teas.

CONTRAINDICATIONS: None known.

St. John's wort *(Hypericum perforatum)*

St. John's wort, although famous for its use in treating depression in modern times, was first used as a topical herb for wound healing and was written about during the early Greek civilization. Many of this herb's properties make it wonderful for topical use: it's astringent, anti-inflammatory, antimicrobial, nervine, and vulnerary. In particular, the infused oil is used for bruises, burns, cuts, skin irritations, sores, and wounds. St. John's wort can also be used as a compress, as a poultice, or in a sitz bath. Its soothing, anti-inflammatory action eases burning and swelling and speeds the healing of perineal tears. The German government allows topical St. John's wort preparations to be labeled for the treatment of first-degree burns, muscular pain, and wounds.

A number of studies of St. John's wort extracts have demonstrated antibacterial activity. For instance, two widely prescribed Russian preparations of St. John's wort have been tested for treatment of *Staphylococcus aureus* infection and been found to be more effective than the drug sulfanilamide.

CONTRAINDICATIONS: St. John's wort is primarily used topically during pregnancy. It can interact with some medications, so check before using.

Strawberry leaves (*Fragaria vesca*)

Strawberry leaves are extremely rich in antioxidants and have a very high vitamin C content. This herb is a mild astringent.

CONTRAINDICATIONS: None known. However, strawberry leaves should not be used by people who are allergic to strawberries.

Tea, black (SEE BLACK TEA, PAGE 52)

Trillium (SEE BETH ROOT, PAGE 51)

Valerian (*Valeriana officinalis*)

Valerian is a wonderful pain reliever. It can also assist with relaxation and sleep. Valerian liniment or extract can be used to massage sore thighs and backs during labor or pregnancy. Although it has been found to slow pre-term labor, valerian will not stop a preterm delivery.

CONTRAINDICATIONS: Although valerian is generally considered safe, it should be used only with professional guidance during pregnancy.

Violet flowers, violet leaves (*Viola odorata*)

As a culinary herb, violet is very safe. In general, it's used to treat colds and coughs and relieve tension and stress.

CONTRAINDICATIONS: None known.

White oak bark (*Quercus robur*)

Anti-inflammatory, antiseptic, and astringent, white oak bark relieves irritation on the surface of tissues because of its numbing action, which can also reduce surface inflammation. In addition, this herb creates a topical barrier against infection, which is an advantage when treating burns and wounds. While white oak bark can be used to soothe perineal discomfort, only a small amount of oak bark is needed in a sitz bath formula; too much can be irritating.

CONTRAINDICATIONS: White oak bark should not be taken internally during pregnancy.

Witch hazel (*Hamamelis virginiana*)

Witch hazel contains tannins, which are astringent and can fight bacteria, reduce irritation and swelling, and repair broken skin when applied topically. Most commercially available witch hazel extracts and other witch hazel products do not contain tannins because they're lost in the distillation process; however, natural witch hazel products can be purchased in some natural food stores or from a local herbalist. Alternatively, Witch Hazel Extract (page 116) can be made at home. The commercial distilled version is still considered beneficial and is worth trying if it's all that's available.

During pregnancy, a strong tea made from the bark and leaves can be used in a sitz bath or compress to treat bacterial vaginosis symptoms. Soothing and cooling, witch hazel mixed with cool water and soaked into a soft cloth can be applied directly to a sore perineum to provide relief. This herb is also great for treating vaginal bruising and varicosities and for slowing bleeding.

CONTRAINDICATIONS: Because witch hazel is an astringent, it should not be taken internally during pregnancy or when nursing.

Yarrow (Achillea millefolium)

Yarrow is considered safe for topical use and is great for treating cuts, scrapes, tears (including perineal tears), varicose veins, and wounds. It's frequently added to sitz baths to be used during the postpartum period.

CONTRAINDICATIONS: Because it can be a uterine stimulant in high doses, it's best to limit its use during the final weeks of pregnancy.

Yellow dock (Rumex crispus)

This herb has long been favored for its ability to improve iron assimilation as well as build blood. It is also reputed to help prevent jaundice in babies.

CONTRAINDICATIONS: Yellow dock can cause loose bowel movements for some people.

HERBS TO AVOID DURING PREGNANCY, LABOR, AND BREASTFEEDING

Use the following herbs only under the direction of an experienced practitioner, if at all. A number of these are safe to use as essential oils but not as fresh or dried herbs.

American pennyroyal (Hedeoma pulegioides)

Physicians, midwives, and other health practitioners know American pennyroyal's well-documented history as a uterine stimulant. As an emmenagogue, this herb stimulates blood flow in the pelvic area and uterus, potentially triggering menstruation. High doses of the herb should be avoided during pregnancy. In addition, there are safety concerns about the use of the essential oil.

Arborvitae *(Thuja occidentalis)*

Also known as western hemlock, arborvitae is a uterine and menstrual stimulant that could cause damage to the fetus. If used without proper guidance, this herb can potentially cause apnea and be lethal.

Autumn crocus *(Colichicum autumnale)*

Autumn crocus can affect cell division, potentially causing birth defects and abnormalities.

Barberry *(Berberis vulgaris)*

Barberry contains high levels of berberine, an alkaloid that can stimulate uterine contractions. It may also interfere with normal bilirubin metabolism in infants, potentially increasing the risk for jaundice and affecting the baby's liver function.

Bladderwrack *(Fucus vesiculosus)*

It is thought that bladderwrack inhibits blood clotting. Taking bladderwrack along with medications that also slow clotting might increase the chances of bruising and bleeding. This herb presents dangers not only to the mother but also to the breastfeeding infant.

Bloodroot *(Sanguinaria canadensis)*

Bloodroot is a uterine stimulant. In addition, quite small doses cause vomiting. This herb contains alkaloids that can potentially cause other issues for the mother and infant. Continual use or overdose of bloodroot can cause abdominal pain, diarrhea, fainting, paralysis, and vision changes.

Broom *(Cytisus scoparius)*

Broom causes uterine contractions so it should be avoided during pregnancy; in parts of Europe it is given after the birth to prevent blood loss. In addition, broom contains a compound called sparteine that slows the cardiac rate and shares some pharmacologic similarities with nicotine; overdose can mimic nicotine poisoning.

Buchu leaves *(Barosma betulina)*

Use of buchu has been linked to miscarriage.

Buckthorn *(Frangula alnus)*

Buckthorn is often used as a laxative. Like most herbs that have a laxative effect, it is not considered safe to use when nursing.

Bugleweed (Lycopus virginicus)

Bugleweed interferes with hormone production in the pituitary gland.

Butterbur (Petasites hybridus)

Butterbur, which is used to treat migraines, contains compounds that might cause birth defects and liver damage.

Cascara sagrada (Rhamnus purshiana)

An extremely strong laxative, cascara sagrada can cause diarrhea and intense abdominal cramping. This herb should not be taken in high doses or for long periods. Some people report cramping and diarrhea even after using small doses.

Chaparral (Larrea tridentate)

Using chaparral when breastfeeding is considered unsafe because it can potentially cause serious liver and kidney problems.

Coltsfoot (Farfarae folium)

Mothers who use coltsfoot run the risk of passing hepatotoxic pyrrolizidine alkaloids, a potentially dangerous compound, to the baby through their breast milk. Even if the coltsfoot remedy is certified to be free of this compound, it's a good idea to just avoid the herb because not enough information is known about its safety.

Cotton root (Gossypium herbaceum)

Cotton root is a uterine stimulant traditionally given to support contractions during a difficult labor. This herb should be used only with professional guidance. I know many midwives who have success with this herb.

Cowslip (Primula veris)

A strong laxative and a uterine stimulant in high doses, cowslip is not used as much in the United States as it is in Europe. Overall, not enough information is known about its effects when used during pregnancy and nursing.

Dong quai (Angelica polymorpha var. sinensis)

Dong quai is a uterine and menstrual stimulant that is not considered safe during pregnancy. Although it is often used after childbirth, it is not recommended when nursing.

Elecampane *(Inula helenium)*

Because of its potential effects on allergies, blood pressure, and blood sugar, elecampane is not considered safe to use when breastfeeding.

Ephedra; Ma huang *(Ephedra sinica)*

Ephedra has been shown to cause anxiety, headache, high blood pressure, irregular heart rhythms, kidney stones, nausea, psychosis, restlessness, sleep problems, stomach irritation, and tremors.

European pennyroyal *(Mentha pulegium)*

European pennyroyal is a uterine stimulant that may contribute to birth defects.

False unicorn root *(Chamaelirium luteum)*

False unicorn root is a hormonal stimulant that should be used only with professional guidance. There is insufficient evidence about this herb's safety.

Ginseng

Many forms of ginseng should not be used during pregnancy or when nursing, or both:

AMERICAN GINSENG *(Panax quinquefolius)*. It has been shown, although not definitively, that American ginseng can potentially affect muscle development in utero, so it is not currently considered safe for pregnancy.

GINSENG *(Panax ginseng)*. The adverse effects of ginseng include nervousness, shakiness, heightened anxiety, insomnia, skin rashes, and diarrhea.

KOREAN GINSENG *(Panax ginseng)*. Clinical reports have shown that use of Korean ginseng during pregnancy can lead to the overstimulation of male sex hormones and, as a result, androgynous babies. If it is used, it should be used for short periods only. Korean ginseng has the same adverse effects as ginseng (see above).

PSEUDOGINSENG *(Panax notoginseng)*. Pseudoginseng is not commonly used in the United States, but it is gaining popularity. It should not be used during pregnancy because it can cause birth defects and possibly miscarriage. Also contraindicated when breastfeeding.

SIBERIAN GINSENG *(Panax ginseng)*. Not considered safe to use during pregnancy, Siberian ginseng can interfere with clotting or clotting disorders. In addition, some research indicates that birth defects are possible with use.

Golden ragwort; Liferoot *(Senecio aureus)*

Also known as liferoot, golden ragwort is a uterine stimulant that also contains toxic chemicals that can cross the placental barrier.

Goldenseal *(Hydrastis canadensis)*

Although safe for topical use, goldenseal should not be taken internally during pregnancy because it is a uterine stimulant and may lead to premature contractions. However, it is safe to use during childbirth. Goldenseal contains berberine, which may interfere with normal bilirubin metabolism in infants, potentially increasing the risk for jaundice and affecting the baby's liver function.

Greater celandine *(Chelidonium majus)*

Greater celandine is a uterine stimulant and can cause premature contractions. Although this herb should not be taken internally when breastfeeding, topical use is safe.

Herb Robert *(Geranium robertianum)*

Not enough information is known about herb Robert.

Juniper *(Juniperus communis)*

Juniper is a uterine stimulant. Although some sources say juniper is safe to use during labor, I would not recommend its use at all during pregnancy. Many safer alternative remedies are available.

Kava kava *(Piper methysticum)*

Kava kava contains chemicals that cause intense relaxation. Because the effects of passing these chemicals to the baby through breast milk are unknown, this herb is not recommended during breastfeeding.

Liferoot (SEE GOLDEN RAGWORT, ABOVE)

Ma huang (SEE EPHEDRA, PAGE 71)

Mistletoe *(Viscum album)*

Mistletoe is a uterine stimulant that also contains potentially toxic constituents that may cross the placental barrier. This herb can be toxic in relatively small doses.

Mugwort *(Artemesia vulgaris)*

Mugwort is a uterine stimulant that may also cause birth defects; some cases of miscarriage have been linked to this herb.

Pennyroyal, American (SEE AMERICAN PENNYROYAL, PAGE 68)

Pennyroyal, European (SEE EUROPEAN PENNYROYAL, PAGE 71)

Periwinkle *(Vinca minor)*

Periwinkle can have negative effects on blood pressure.

Peruvian bark *(Cinchona officinalis)*

When used in excess, Peruvian bark can be toxic and cause blindness and coma. This herb is often used to treat malaria and should be used only with professional guidance.

Poke root *(Phytolacca decandra)*

Poke root can cause birth defects and can potentially be quite toxic. If this herb is used improperly, ingestion can lead to diarrhea, difficulty breathing, confusion, nausea, rapid heart rate, rapid loss of blood pressure, vomiting, and possibly even death.

Pulsatilla *(Anemone pulsatilla)*

Pulsatilla, which stimulates menstruation, is often found in homeopathic remedies.

Rhubarb *(Rheum rhabarbarum)*

Rhubarb is often used as a laxative. Like most herbs that have a laxative effect, it is not considered safe to use when breastfeeding.

Rue *(Ruta graveolens)*

Rue has a long history of use. It is a uterine and menstrual stimulant and has been known to cause premature contractions.

Sassafras *(Sassafras albidum)*

Sassafras is a uterine stimulant that may also cause birth defects. In addition, it is a documented abortifacient and emmenagogue.

Southernwood *(Artemisia abrotanum)*

Southernwood is a uterine stimulant that may also cause birth defects. It should be used during pregnancy only with professional guidance.

Squill *(Urginea maritima)*

Rarely used in the United States, squill is a uterine stimulant that may also cause birth defects.

Star anise *(Illicium verum)*

Star anise may be contaminated with Japanese star anise, a known neurotoxin. In addition, adverse reactions in children have been recorded.

Tansy *(Tanacetum vulgare)*

Tansy is a uterine stimulant that may also cause birth defects. Although it is not commonly used in modern herbalism, it may be used to stimulate the uterus or expel worms.

Uva ursi *(Arctostaphylos uva ursi)*

Uva ursi is not safe for people who have high blood pressure.

Vervain *(Verbena officinalis)*

Vervain is a potential uterine stimulant in high doses, but it is generally safe to use during labor. Because there is some evidence that it can limit iron absorption in infants, it should not be used when breastfeeding.

Western hemlock (SEE ARBORVITAE, PAGE 69)

Wild lettuce *(Lactuca virosa)*

Wild lettuce can have a narcotic effect and is not well researched in terms of safety.

Wood betony *(Stachys officinalis)*

Wood betony is not well researched.

Wormwood *(Artemisia absinthium)*

Wormwood is an abortifacient that may also cause birth defects. It should be used during pregnancy only with professional guidance.

HERBS THAT ARE SAFE FOR CULINARY USE

A number of the following herbs will cause uterine contractions or promote bleeding if taken internally in large amounts. They also may pass on undesirable substances in breast milk. However, they are safe for culinary use. In addition, the small amounts used in personal care products are generally safe, as are some topical applications.

Celery seeds *(Apium graveolens)*

Chiles *(Capsicum)*

Lesser galangal *(Alpinia officinarum)*

Lovage *(Levisticum officinale)*

Marjoram *(Origanum majorana)*

Myrrh *(Commiphora myrrha)*

Nutmeg *(Myristica fragrans)*

Oregano *(Origanum vulgare, Origanum onites, Origanum syriacum)*

Saffron *(Crocus sativus)*

Sage *(Salvia officinalis)*

Sorrel *(Rumex acetosa)*

Turmeric *(Curcuma longa)*

White horehound *(Marrubium vulgare)*

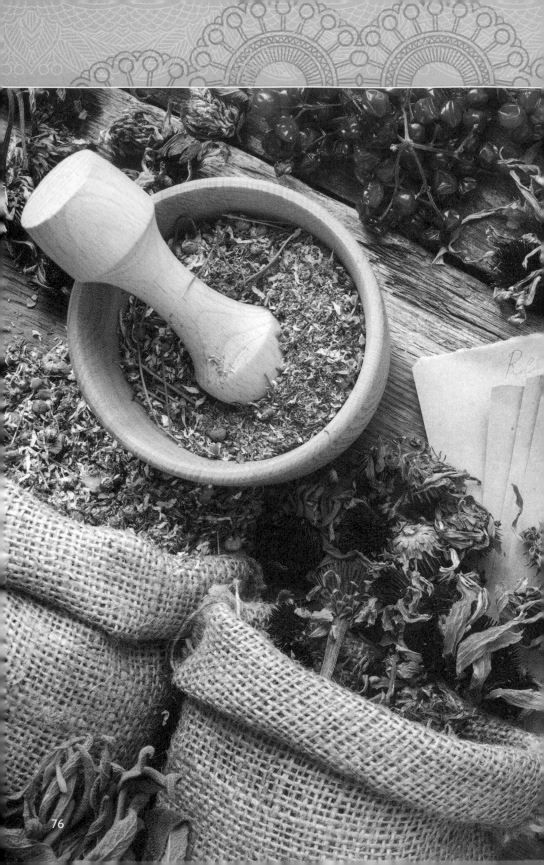

Making Your Own Aromatherapy and Herbal Remedies

These days, aromatherapy and prepared herbal remedies are sold almost everywhere, including big-box discount stores, natural food stores, pharmacies, supermarkets, and online. Instead of buying commercially made remedies, why not try your hand at making your own? Once you have the right ingredients and equipment, the processes are quite easy.

Most homemade aromatherapy remedies are in the form of body sprays, room sprays, bath oils, massage oils, diffuser blends, creams, lotions, liniments, and salves. All aromatherapy remedies are used topically or inhaled; essential oils and aromatherapy remedies should never be ingested. General directions for making these products are provided in "Basic Methods for Making Aromatherapy Remedies," which follows.

Homemade herbal remedies can take the form of decoctions, infusions, extracts, tinctures, lozenges, and syrups, which are all taken internally. You can also make liniments, salves, compresses, poultices, and plasters, which are all used topically. General directions for making these items are provided in "Basic Methods for Making Herbal Remedies" (page 81).

My aromatherapy remedies and herbal remedies for pregnancy, labor, and the postpartum period are provided in chapters 6, 7, and 8. These are written as easy-to-follow recipes. Because many of the basic methods in this chapter provide information that is essential for making the specific remedies, you'll often be referred back to them.

BASIC METHODS FOR MAKING AROMATHERAPY REMEDIES

Before trying the remedies (pages 89 to 169) for any aromatherapy application, review the following section to become familiar with the basic methods. My aromatherapy remedies in chapters 6, 7, and 8 provide more specifics, such as the types and amounts of the ingredients and usage instructions.

Making Body Sprays with Essential Oils

To make a body spray, combine essential oils with a food-grade alcohol, such as vodka, or water in a clean glass or metal spray bottle. A typical formula is to put 30 to 40 drops of essential oils in a 4-ounce glass spray bottle, but my remedies may vary. Add enough vodka or water to fill the bottle. Put the spray cap on the bottle and shake well to combine.

NOTE: Alcohol, such as vodka, acts as a preservative.

Making Room Sprays with Essential Oils

Although they are similar to body sprays, room sprays tend to be more concentrated. To make a room spray, combine essential oils with a food-grade alcohol, such as vodka, or water in a clean glass or metal spray bottle that can be set to distribute a fine mist. A typical formula is to put about 40 drops of essential oils in a 4-ounce or 5-ounce glass spray bottle, but my remedies may vary. Add enough vodka or water to fill the bottle. Put the spray cap on the bottle and shake well to combine.

CAUTION: Never direct a room spray directly at yourself.

NOTE: Alcohol, such as vodka, acts as a preservative.

Making Bath Oils with Essential Oils

An easy way to enjoy aromatherapy is to add essential oils to a bath. All you need per bath is 1 teaspoon to 1 tablespoon of an essential oil or blend. A little oil goes a really long way. Make sure the essential oil or blend is adequately dispersed in the water.

When you want to design your own essential oil blends for use in aromatherapy and are not following one of my remedies, consider the following guidelines:

- First determine the types of essential oils that may be useful by researching various oils and their therapeutic effects. List the primary results you desire, such as pain reduction, and the supportive actions you desire, such as mood enhancement. Then select the essential oils that meet your needs.

- Use your research to determine the number of drops of each essential oil to start with.

- Put the appropriate number of essential oil drops in a clean dropper bottle or jar using a dropper or pipette. Start with equal amounts of the essential oils and increase them one at a time if desired. Put the cap on tightly and gently swish the bottle in a circular motion to mix. Remove the cap to test the fragrance and effect.

- If you have them, use scent strips (neutral blotter strips that are used for testing a fragrance) to test the blend. Put a few drops on a strip and smell away.

- When you're ready to use the essential oil blend, add the carrier oil (see box, page 14).

Making Blended and Massage Oils with Essential Oils

Blended and massage oils are made with a carrier oil (see box, page 14) and essential oils. When making one of my remedies, put all the ingredients in a clean glass bottle, put the cap on tightly, and swish gently to combine. To design your own massage oil, add a few drops of essential oils per 1 tablespoon of carrier oil. Test before using. If the massage oil blend is too strong, add more carrier oil to dilute it. If the massage oil isn't potent enough, add a few more drops of essential oil. After mixing, all massage oils should be transferred to a clean, dry glass bottle. Put the cap on tightly and store in a dry place.

Making Diffuser Blends with Essential Oils

When making one of my diffuser blend remedies, put all the ingredients in a clean glass jar, put the lid on tightly, and swish gently to combine. In addition, many of the remedies for blended and massage oils in this book can be used as diffuser blends if the carrier oil is omitted. If you'd like to design your own, following are a few popular essential oils to use in diffuser blends:

- Cedarwood, clary sage, lavender, Roman chamomile, and tangerine can help to relieve stress.

- Cedarwood, clary sage, frankincense, lavender, Roman chamomile, rosewood, sandalwood, tangerine, and ylang-ylang can help relieve tension.

NOTE: It's critical to check the diffuser manufacturer's instructions when using essential oil blends in a diffuser; one important consideration is the amount of oil that can be safely used in the diffuser at one time. The recommended diffuser blends in this book may produce amounts that are too great to be diffused at one time.

Making Creams and Lotions with Essential Oils

Start with a favorite cream or lotion, preferably unscented, and thoroughly mix in the essential oil or blend. A typical formula is to combine 15 to 30 drops of essential oils with 1 ounce of cream or lotion, but my remedies may vary. Test before using. The fatty base of some creams or lotions may make an essential oil feel stronger; if so, try adding a bit more cream or lotion to dilute. Store creams and lotions in a tightly sealed glass bottle or jar.

Making Liniments with Essential Oils

Liniments are made with food-grade alcohol, such as vodka, or witch hazel and essential oils. When making one of my remedies, put all the ingredients in a clean glass bottle, put the cap on tightly, and shake well to combine. Let steep as directed. For your own blend, use 1 teaspoon of essential oil (such as eucalyptus or peppermint) per ½ cup of vodka and let steep for at least 14 days.

CAUTION: Do not use rubbing alcohol to make a liniment since it can irritate the skin, eyes, and mucous membranes.

Making Salves with Essential Oils

Salves are made with both a carrier oil (see box, page 14) and a hard wax or oil, such as beeswax, candelilla wax, or coconut oil. A typical formula to make 2 cups of salve is to combine 2 cups of carrier oil and 3 tablespoons of wax with the desired number of essential oil drops, although my remedies vary and often don't yield this volume.

Put the carrier oil and wax in a small saucepan and warm over low heat, stirring until all the wax is melted. Stir in the essential oils. Pour into a clean glass bottle or salve jar. Test the salve when it cools. If it seems too hard, repeat the process and add more drops of essential oil. Similarly, if it seems too soft, add more wax. Store in a tightly sealed glass bottle or salve jar. Following are examples of essential oils that work well in salves:

- Bergamot, chamomile (German and Roman), frankincense, and neroli essential oils can help relieve stress.
- Black pepper, clary sage, and Roman chamomile essential oils are good for muscle aches and pains.
- Lavender, palmarosa, and rosewood essential oils have healing properties.

BASIC METHODS FOR MAKING HERBAL REMEDIES

Before trying the remedies for any herbal application, review this section to become familiar with the basic methods. My herbal remedies in chapters 6, 7, and 8 provide more specifics, such as the types and amounts of the ingredients and usage instructions.

Making Decoctions with Herbs

Decoctions are used to make teas as well as compresses and liniments. A typical formula is to put 1 to 2 tablespoons of herbs and 1 cup of water in a saucepan over medium heat, cover, and let simmer for 20 minutes. Remove from the heat and let steep for 20 to 30 minutes. (I like to let my decoctions steep for a generous amount of time—a few hours sometimes—because I suggest them for so many tonic and medicinal uses.) Strain the decoction into a clean, dry jar and put the lid on tightly. Store decoctions in the refrigerator or a cool place. Decoctions don't keep well, so plan to use them within 48 hours of preparation.

Making Infusions (Teas and Infused Oils) with Herbs

HERBAL TEA. Herbal teas can be made using one or more herbs. When combining dried herbs to make an herbal blend that will yield multiple cups of tea, put the herbs in a clean glass jar and mix until well combined. Put the lid on the jar and close it tightly.

A typical formula for making herbal tea is to use 1 to 2 teaspoons of a dried herb (or an herbal blend) per 1 cup of boiling water. Let steep for 10 to 20 minutes, strain, and discard the herbs. Stored in a covered pitcher in the refrigerator, prepared herbal tea will keep for 1 to 2 days.

INFUSED OILS. Infused oils are popular because they're so concentrated with healing compounds. As a bonus, infused oils are easy to make. Simply put the fresh or dried herbs in a clean, sterilized jar, cover the herbs with oil, and put the lid on the jar. I prefer to use olive oil, although sunflower oil and grapeseed oil can also be used if you have them on hand. Some herbalists follow formulas and ratios of herbs to oil, but I just pack the jar with herbs and cover them completely with oil. As a result, my oils come out richly colored. For example, St. John's wort infused oil is bright red, lavender-infused oil is purple, and comfrey- or plantain-infused oils are spring green.

Once the herbs and oil are in the jar, there are a couple of ways to steep an infusion. One method is to put the jar in the sunshine for two weeks, then strain the oil through a piece of cheesecloth into a clean, dry jar. (For really potent oil, repeat the process, reusing the infused oil in a jar full of fresh herbs.) Put the lid on tightly and store the jar in a dry, cool place. This method is particularly good for making colorful oils with rose hips and St. John's wort because the long steeping time extracts more bioflavonoids and other active constituents.

A second method is to put the jar containing the herbs and oil in simmering water in a slow cooker. The water level should be about one inch below the jar's lid. Keep an eye on the water level and don't let it go down. Maintain it by refilling with boiling water as needed. After four hours, remove the jar from the slow cooker. When the jar is cool enough to handle, strain the infused oil through a piece of cheesecloth into a clean, dry jar. Put the lid on tightly and store the jar in a dry, cool place.

You can also use a double boiler to make an infusion. Put the herbs in the top of the double boiler until it is one-half to three-quarters full. Cover the herbs with vegetable oil. Put water in the bottom of the double boiler, insert the top, cover, and heat over medium heat until the water is gently simmering. If necessary, decrease the heat so the water stays at a gentle simmer for about three hours. Remove from the heat and let cool. Strain through a piece of cheesecloth or muslin into a clean jar and put the lid on tightly. Discard the herbs. For some additional, extra-strong energy, put infused oils under the light of a full moon for one night.

Infused oils will keep for up to two years. Discard if mold forms.

Making Extracts with Herbs

An extract is similar to a tincture (see opposite page) in that it contains an herb's active ingredients in a concentrated form. The herb is extracted by soaking it for a long period in alcohol or pure vegetable glycerin. Glycerin is a popular choice when making remedies for pregnant women because it contains no alcohol. But even when an extract is made with alcohol, one dose of finished extract contains very little alcohol. **Note:** If you use glycerin, you must use dried, not fresh, herbs.

To make an extract, put the dried or fresh herbs in a clean, sterilized, and dry jar. Cover dried herbs with the alcohol (or glycerin) by two inches and fresh herbs with alcohol by one inch. (Dried herbs absorb more liquid and expand.) Put the lid on the jar and close tightly. Let it sit in the sunlight for a few days. For extra potency, put the jar under a full moon all night or in the sun all afternoon. (Among herbalists, it is a time-honored tradition to begin making extracts on the eve of the new moon and strain on the full moon. The waxing powers of the moon extract the most therapeutic agents from the herbs.)

Store the jar in a cupboard or other dark place and let the extract steep for two weeks. It will be saturated with color from the herbs. Strain it through a piece of cheesecloth or muslin into a sterile glass jar. Squeeze or press the soaked herbs, extracting as much of the liquid as possible. Discard the herbs. Put the lid on the jar and label it with the names of the herbs and the date. The extract is now ready to use.

Always store extracts in a dry, dark place. Alcohol extracts will keep for two to five years; glycerin extracts will keep for one to three years.

NOTE: The terms "extract" and "tincture" are often, and inaccurately, inter-changed. Most extracts are 40 percent alcohol, whereas tinctures may have the same alcohol content but not as much of the herb.

Making Tinctures with Herbs

Making tinctures is actually pretty simple. However, if you want the variety that most people prefer to have in a well-stocked medicine chest, it's probably cheaper to buy tinctures.

To make a tincture, put the fresh or dried herbs in a widemouthed jar (the size depends on how much tincture you want to make). I usually fill a quart jar until the herbs are two inches from the top. Completely cover the herbs with 80- to 100-proof vodka, brandy, or rum. I have even used twenty-year-old Irish whiskey.

A good ratio to follow is one part dried herbs to five parts alcohol or one part fresh herbs to three parts alcohol. Cover dried herbs with the alcohol by two inches and fresh herbs by one inch. (Dried herbs absorb more liquid and expand.) Put the lid on the jar and close it tightly. Put the jar in a dark place, such as a cabinet or closet, to let the tincture steep. Shake the jar gently every day.

The tincture will be ready in four to eight weeks. Strain the liquid through a piece of cheesecloth or muslin into a sterile, dark glass tincture bottle. Squeeze or press the soaked herbs, extracting as much of the liquid as possible. Discard the herbs. Put the cap on the bottle and label it with the name of the herbs and the date. The tincture is now ready to use. Tinctures will keep for several months to several years when stored in dark glass bottles in a cool place away from sunlight.

Commercial tinctures are labeled with the recommended dosage, usually 10 to 30 drops orally, three times per day. However, tincture dosages are best determined individually based on the severity of the illness and the strength of the herb. To determine the correct dose, follow the dosage instructions in my remedies (see pages 89 to 169), consult a professional herbalist, or rely on a couple of good reference books.

NOTE: The terms "extract" and "tincture" are often, and inaccurately, interchanged. Most extracts are 40 percent alcohol, whereas tinctures may have the same alcohol content but not as much of the herb.

Making Lozenges with Herbs

Lozenges are made with powdered herbs, which can be purchased or made from dried herbs. An easy way to grind dried herbs into powder is to use a coffee grinder.

To make lozenges, put the powdered herbs in a large bowl. Add a small amount of honey and a little water and stir. Keep stirring, adding water a little at a time until the mixture reaches a dough-like consistency. It will be sticky because of the honey. With your hands, roll the dough into balls or disks about one-half to three-quarters inch in diameter. Roll the balls in ground carob or slippery elm, then put them on baking sheets. Set them on the kitchen counter if it's a warm, dry day or put them in the oven at the lowest temperature setting (in a gas oven, heat from the pilot light will be sufficient). Dry the lozenges completely (this will take thirty to sixty minutes) and let them cool completely. The lozenges can also be dried in a food dehydrator at 110 to 115 degrees F for ten to forty-eight hours. The dehydration time will depend on how moist the dough is. I like the Excalibur dehydrator, but you can find dehydrators at most big-box stores, natural food stores, and online.

Making Syrups with Herbs

Many prepared herb-based syrups are available at natural food stores. Instructions for their use and storage are provided on the label. My remedy for Iron-Rich Syrup (page 92) provides an example of how to simmer herbs in water for several hours and then cook down the mixture into a reduction. Although Iron-Rich Syrup keeps in the refrigerator for two weeks, most homemade herbal syrups should keep for one month in the refrigerator. However, if it contains glycerin or alcohol, the syrup will keep for six months. Discard syrups if mold appears.

Making Liniments with Herbs

To make one of my favorite liniments, put 4 ounces of fresh or dried peppermint leaves and 4 ounces of fresh or dried eucalyptus leaves in a 16-ounce jar. Cover the herbs with 2 cups of vodka or vinegar. Let steep in a dry place for 14 days and shake the contents twice a day. For added potency, you can also add a few drops of essential oil, such as eucalyptus or peppermint, if you like.

CAUTION: Do not use rubbing alcohol to make a liniment since it can irritate the skin, eyes, and mucous membranes.

Making Salves with Herbs

Making your own salve may sound laborious, but it's not. The simple formula is to melt grated beeswax, candelilla wax, or coconut oil with a carrier oil (see box, page 14) in a double boiler, stir in herb-infused oils, pour the mixture into glass salve pots or small glass jars, and let it cool and solidify. Test the salve before using. If it's too hard, melt it again and add more carrier oil; if it's too soft, melt it and add more grated beeswax. To find sources for beeswax and salve jars, see Suppliers, page 174.

If you'd like to try your hand at making salves, start with some basic ones that can be used for many common conditions. Following is a list of frequently used salves:

- Calendula salve is gentle and versatile; it is excellent for eczema, diaper rash, and dry, cracked skin.
- Comfrey salve cools inflamed skin and helps heal rashes and other skin problems.
- Plantain salve has strongly astringent and soothing properties and helps to relieve the pain of wounds, stings, and insect bites. In addition, it helps to stop bleeding.

Making Compresses with Herbs

Cold compresses are useful for small bruises and other minor boo-boos. The simple formula for making a cold compress is to put cold water in a bowl, mix in the herb, and soak a cloth in the water. When I need to make a compress quickly, I soak the cloth in one or more herbal extracts. Depending on how strong I want to make the compress, I may or may not dilute the herbal extracts.

A different type of compress is called a fomentation, which is a hot compress and an especially good treatment for pain and swelling. They are great to use during labor.

To make a fomentation, make a hot herbal tea as an infusion (see page 81) and put it in a bowl. Soak a soft cloth, such as a cloth diaper or washcloth, in the infusion. Squeeze out some of the excess liquid; the cloth should be very wet but not dripping. Apply the cloth as hot as can be tolerated. To hold in the heat, cover the cloth with a piece of flannel or another cloth or towel that has been warmed. (Microwave ovens can be used to heat cloth and may be accessible at a birth center or hospital. Electric or gas ovens that are set on low heat can work as well.) Reapply the fomentation as needed.

Making Poultices with Herbs

A poultice is similar to a compress except that fresh herbs are used instead of decoctions or infusions. Poultices are considered more "active" than compresses. They are used to stimulate circulation, ease aches and pains, or draw impurities from the body through the skin; therefore, they need to remain in place for a few hours at a time.

There are several ways that you can make a poultice. The simplest method is to mash or crush the fresh herbs with a rolling pin on a clean cloth and fold up the cloth so the herbs are wrapped inside. Apply the poultice to the affected area and cover it with another cloth to hold in body heat.

To make a steamed poultice, mash the fresh herbs with a mortar and pestle or process them in a food processor to make a pulp. Heat the pulp in a colander over boiling water or in a steamer. Alternatively, mix it with a small amount of boiling water. Remove from the heat and let the pulp cool until it is still very warm but can be handled, about ten minutes. Apply the pulp directly to the skin as hot as can be tolerated, holding it in place with a gauze bandage. A hot water bottle can be held against the bandage to keep the poultice warm. As soon as the steamed poultice cools, apply another.

To make a steamed poultice quickly, put enough herbs to cover the affected area in a small saucepan and just cover with water. Simmer for two minutes. Drain off the water and squeeze out the excess liquid. To apply the poultice, rub a little vegetable oil on the skin in the affected area to prevent the poultice from sticking and apply the warm herbs directly to the oiled skin. Hold the poultice in place using strips of gauze or cotton fabric and leave it in place for two to three hours. Wrapping the poultice in wool cloth will keep it warm longer. Change the poultice when it cools.

Making Plasters with Herbs

A plaster is similar to a poultice, but dried herbs are typically used. Grind the dried herbs into a powder using a blender, food processor, or mortar and pestle. Make a paste by mixing one tablespoon of the powdered herbs with a little boiling water or hot cider vinegar. Smear the herb paste on a piece of wool or gauze, cover it with another piece of wool or gauze, and apply this plaster, or "sandwich," to the skin. If you're using fresh herbs for plasters, pulverize them in a food processor or a blender. Alternatively, finely chop or mash them by hand.

Depending on the herbs used, plasters can be left in place for several hours, even overnight. Leave plasters in place for less time, however, when using herbs that could irritate the skin, such as garlic or horseradish.

Plasters are helpful for treating general aches and pains, arthritis, back pain, chronic injuries, frozen shoulders, muscle pains and strains, tennis elbow, and sciatica. They should not be used on open wounds, damaged skin, or irritated skin. And they should not be used on children age two and younger.

Making a Sitz Bath with Herbs

A sitz bath is a localized bath, taken in a bathtub or a pan designed to fit over the commode, in which you sit in warm water that covers the buttocks and hips. This bath is beneficial for any issue that requires the medicinal application of herbs to the area between the vagina and anus. Sitting in warm water allows more blood to reach the area, promoting healing and alleviating discomfort. Sitz baths have long been used to treat hemorrhoids and postpartum pain and swelling.

To make a typical sitz bath, boil 1 gallon of water, add 2 to 3 cups of dried herbs, and let steep for 30 minutes. Fill a sitz bath pan or a regular bathtub with a few inches of warm water, and mix the herbal blend into the water. Sit in the sitz bath for 20 minutes. Rinse off with warm water after your bath and dry yourself gently.

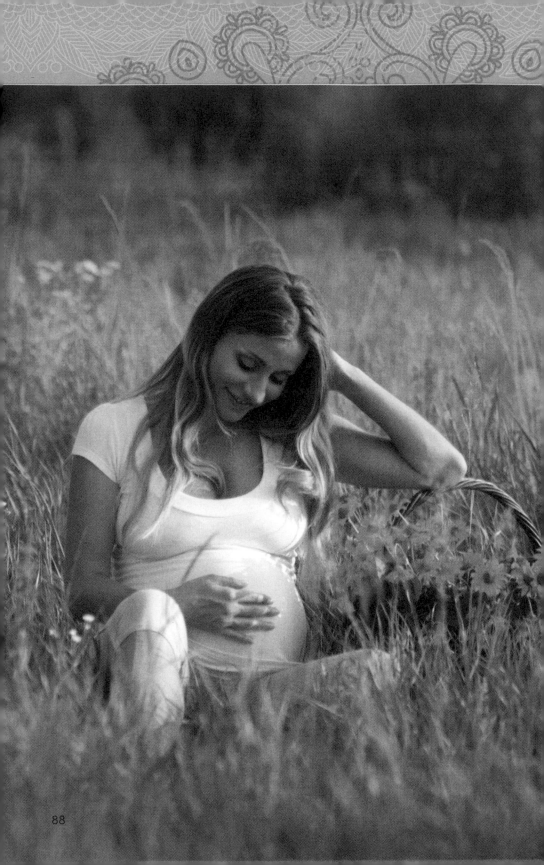

Remedies for Pregnancy

This chapter features aromatherapy and herbal remedies for the prenatal period, which extends from conception to labor. This chapter is organized alphabetically by the names of health issues pregnant women experience. For most issues, multiple remedies are suggested. All these remedies are specifically recommended for the prenatal period and are generally considered safe to use during pregnancy.

Some of the issues listed here do not occur frequently, but others are so common that most mothers have had them and can name friends who have had them as well. Women in conversation often bond sharing stories of their pregnancies with each other. In a way, the health challenges of pregnancy are the growing pains on the path to motherhood. The good news is that aromatherapy and herbal remedies provide welcome solutions and relief.

When you are pregnant or breastfeeding, you naturally care deeply about what goes into your body and your baby's body. It is essential that before you use any remedy, natural or not, you research it first. Seek professional advice if you need to. Always discuss any remedies that you use with your care provider.

GENERAL PREGNANCY SUPPORT

The following nutritious teas are great choices for supporting your health during pregnancy. In addition to providing a healthful boost, delicious herbal teas encourage you to slow down, have a seat, and savor a cup.

Pregnancy Tea 1

YIELD: 2 CUPS DRIED TEA

½ cup **dried nettles**
½ cup **dried peach leaves**
½ cup **dried peppermint leaves**
½ cup **dried raspberry leaves**

Follow the method for making herbal teas as infusions, page 81. Let steep for 15 to 30 minutes.

DOSAGE INSTRUCTIONS: Drink 2 to 3 cups per day.

Pregnancy Tea 2

YIELD: 3 CUPS DRIED TEA

1 cup **dried nettles**
1 cup **dried raspberry leaves**
½ cup **dried alfalfa leaves**
½ cup **dried rose hips**

Follow the method for making herbal teas as infusions, page 81. Let steep for 15 to 30 minutes.

DOSAGE INSTRUCTIONS: Drink 2 to 3 cups per day.

Pregnancy Tea 3

YIELD: 3 CUPS DRIED TEA

1 cup	**dried alfalfa leaves**
1 cup	**dried nettles**
1 cup	**dried raspberry leaves**

Follow the method for making herbal teas as infusions, page 81. Let steep for 20 to 30 minutes.

DOSAGE INSTRUCTIONS: Drink 2 to 3 cups per day.

ANEMIA

Anemia is a condition that occurs when the iron levels in your blood are low. This can be determined by a simple blood test. Iron helps your red blood cells carry oxygen to all parts of your body and especially critical during pregnancy, when your daily iron needs increase from 18 to 27 milligrams. Some iron-rich herbs are dandelion leaves, dried nettles, raspberry leaves, and yellow dock.

Following are the signs and symptoms of anemia:

- appetite loss
- dizzines
- drowsiness
- fatigue
- headaches
- malaise
- nausea and vomiting
- skin pallor
- sore tongue
- pale fingernail beds
- pale mucous membranes

Iron-Rich Tea

YIELD: ABOUT 8 CUPS PREPARED TEA

8 cups	**water**
3 tablespoons	**dried nettles**
2 tablespoons	**dried raspberry leaves**
1 tablespoon	**dried dandelion leaves**
1 tablespoon	**diced seeded rose hips**

Pour the water into a medium saucepan and heat over medium heat until the water just begins to boil. Remove from the heat and stir in the nettles, raspberry leaves, dandelion leaves, and rose hips. Let steep, covered, for 30 minutes before drinking.

DOSAGE INSTRUCTIONS: Drink 3 to 5 cups per day.

Iron-Rich Tincture

YIELD: VARIABLE

3 tablespoons	**dried nettles**
2 tablespoons	**dried raspberry leaves**
1 tablespoon	**dried dandelion leaves**
1 tablespoon	**diced seeded rose hips**

Follow the method for making tinctures, page 83, using enough alcohol to cover the herbs with 1 to 2 inches to spare. When the herbs absorb the alcohol, you may need to add more alcohol to maintain a level 1 to 2 inches above the herbs. Let steep for 3 to 6 weeks.

DOSAGE INSTRUCTIONS: Take 20 to 30 drops orally, 2 to 3 times per day.

Iron-Rich Syrup

YIELD: ABOUT 7 CUPS

6 cups	**water**
½ ounce	**dried dandelion root**
½ ounce	**dried rose hips**
½ ounce	**dried yellow dock root**
¾ cup	**blackstrap molasses**

Put the water, dandelion root, rose hips, and yellow dock root in a medium saucepan over high heat. Bring to a boil, then decrease the heat to low. Cover and let simmer for 4½ hours, monitoring it occasionally.

Strain the liquid into another medium saucepan. Simmer on low heat, uncovered, until the liquid is reduced to 1½ cups, 1 to 2 hours. Stir in the molasses until well incorporated. Pour into a clean glass canning jar, allow to cool to room temperature, and put the lid on tightly. Stored in the refrigerator, the syrup will keep for 2 weeks.

DOSAGE INSTRUCTIONS: Take 1 to 2 tablespoons daily. Try stirring Iron-Rich Syrup into warm tea, oatmeal, or a smoothie.

NOTE: The body absorbs iron best when it is consumed with foods rich in vitamin C, such as citrus fruits. Blackstrap molasses is the dark liquid by-product that results when sugarcane is refined into white sugar. It is highly concentrated and rich in nutrients, including iron (see box, opposite page). Adding molasses can be a simple and easy way to boost your nutritional intake. For example, blackstrap molasses can be used to sweeten smoothies and other dishes. In addition to being nutritious, blackstrap molasses has an advantage over iron

NUTRIENTS IN BLACKSTRAP MOLASSES

The following nutrients are found in 2 teaspoons (13.67 grams) of molasses, which has 32 calories.

NUTRIENT	PERCENTAGE OF DAILY VALUE
Manganese	18
Copper	14
Iron	13.2
Calcium	11.7
Potassium	9.7
Magnesium	7.3
Vitamin B_6	5

supplements because it does not promote constipation like an iron supplement can.

ANXIETY

Anxiety is becoming a more common diagnosis among women given today's stressful lifestyles. Anxiety is a general term that is used to describe feeling anxious, fearful, nervous, apprehensive, and worried. When women are pregnant, their hormones, protective instincts, and financial and other practical concerns about impending parenthood can cause anxiety. Indeed, having a baby on the way can produce anxiety in both parents.

Antianxiety medications are widely available; however, limited information is available about how prescription drugs, including antianxiety medications, affect women during pregnancy. It's common for women to discontinue antianxiety medications when they are pregnant. The downside to doing this is that pregnant women may experience worsening anxiety symptoms; for many, the first trimester can be especially difficult.

With or without the aid of medication, you can relieve anxiety by relaxing, meditating, taking walks, and doing yoga. Try to do something enjoyable every day, such as having lunch with friends or simply reading a joke online.

Aromatherapy remedies, from diffuser blends to room sprays to bath oils, can be particularly calming. You may notice that all the essential oils featured in the following antianxiety remedies are from the citrus family. I love these oils because they bring calm and sunshine into any room. Their aromas are warm, cheery, and comforting.

In addition to using aromatherapy, drinking herbal teas is also an excellent choice. The simple act of drinking a cup of hot tea encourages you to slow down and relax. Make teatime a slow, gentle time for yourself. Take a seat, breathe deeply, sip your tea, and enjoy a few moments of quiet for yourself. This can decrease anxiety levels and boost your overall mood.

Diffuser Blend for Anxiety

YIELD: 20 DROPS

10 drops	**neroli essential oil**
5 drops	**bergamot essential oil**
5 drops	**ylang-ylang essential oil**

Follow the method for making diffuser blends, page 79.

USAGE INSTRUCTIONS: Follow the manufacturer's instructions for using your model of diffuser.

Room Spray for Anxiety 1

YIELD: ABOUT 6 OUNCES

5 ounces	**water**
1 ounce	**80-proof vodka**
20 drops	**grapefruit essential oil**
10 drops	**lavender essential oil**
10 drops	**ylang-ylang essential oil**

Follow the method for making room sprays, page 78.

Room Spray for Anxiety 2

YIELD: ABOUT 6 OUNCES

5 ounces	**water**
1 ounce	**80-proof vodka**
10 drops	**mandarin essential oil**
10 drops	**sweet orange essential oil**
10 drops	**tangerine essential oil**

Follow the method for making room sprays, page 78.

Anxiety-Relief Bath Oil

YIELD: ABOUT 1 OUNCE

1 ounce	**carrier oil** (see note)
5 drops	**sandalwood essential oil**
2 drops	**mandarin essential oil**

Follow the method for making bath oils, page 78.

USAGE INSTRUCTIONS: Add ½ teaspoon to the bath water and distribute well. While in the tub, let the bath wash away worries and stress.

CAUTION: Bath oil can cause a slippery tub, so be careful.

NOTE: When making this bath oil, I choose a carrier oil based on the season. In the winter I use a thicker oil, such as olive oil or warmed coconut oil, to really soothe dry skin; in the summer, I use a lighter oil, such as apricot kernel oil or grapeseed oil.

Antianxiety Infusion

YIELD: 3 TABLESPOONS DRIED TEA

1 tablespoon	**dried lemon balm leaves**
1 tablespoon	**dried nettle leaves**
1 tablespoon	**dried raspberry leaves**

Follow the method for making infusions, page 81.

DOSAGE INSTRUCTIONS: Drink 2 to 3 cups per day.

NOTE: This remedy is great for moms who are past the first trimester and can provide comfort during the postpartum period.

Easy Antianxiety Tea

YIELD: ABOUT 1 QUART

¼ cup	**chopped fresh lemon balm leaves**
¼ cup	**dried milky oats**
1 quart	**water, boiling hot**

Put the lemon balm and milky oats in a quart jar and pour the water over the herbs. Let steep for 20 minutes.

DOSAGE INSTRUCTIONS: Drink 2 to 3 cups per day.

NOTE: Serve hot or chilled.

BACKACHE

There are many causes of backache, such as an injury, a slipped or herniated disc, arthritis, osteoporosis, overweight, urinary tract infections, sitting or walking improperly, and even stress. During pregnancy, the changing and expanding center of gravity in the body can be a source of back pain. Most backaches are linked to strained muscles in the lower back; we often use these muscles without thinking about how our twists and turns can affect the lower back.

The purpose of herbal remedies is to treat the cause of the backache, relieve the pain, promote back health and healing, and avoid reinjury. Three remedies that can bring relief include massages with essential oils, baths with essential oils, and liniments applied directly to the affected area. Some essential oils that are particularly good for treating back pain include chamomile, lavender, sandalwood, spearmint, and vetiver.

Preventing back injuries is an important part of avoiding backaches. Improper lifting causes a lot of backaches. If you are at a job while pregnant, talk to your care provider about specific lifting guidelines for your pregnancy and postpartum period.

If you strain your back, do not immediately slip into a hot bath, thinking it will relax you. This can cause strained muscles to swell and make matters worse. Wait twenty-four hours before you take a hot bath or apply any heat. If your back is just sore from the excessive weight of pregnancy, enjoy a soothing bath whenever it's needed. Treat your back with care and listen to your pain.

Backache Massage Oil

YIELD: ABOUT 2 OUNCES

2 ounces	**St. John's wort infused oil**
5 drops	**vetiver essential oil**
3 drops	**lavender essential oil**
1 drop	**sandalwood essential oil**

Follow the method for making blended and massage oils, page 79.

APPLICATION INSTRUCTIONS: Shake well before using. Massage into the back as needed.

Backache Bath Oil

YIELD: ENOUGH FOR 1 BATH

lavender essential oil

niaouli essential oil

Roman chamomile essential oil

spearmint essential oil

vetiver essential oil

Draw a warm bath. Add up to 10 drops of the above essential oils in any combination. Do not exceed 10 drops. Experiment to find a combination that smells great to you, fosters relaxation, and relieves tension.

VARIATIONS: Pairings that work wonderfully together include lavender and niaouli, lavender and spearmint, lavender and vetiver, and Roman chamomile and vetiver.

Essential Oil Back Liniment

YIELD: ABOUT 3 OUNCES

3 ounces	vodka
10 drops	lavender essential oil
10 drops	spearmint essential oil
5 drops	chamomile essential oil

Follow the method for making liniments, page 80.

APPLICATION INSTRUCTIONS: Shake well before using. Apply directly to the affected area as needed.

NOTE: If this blend is not strong enough, try adding 3 more drops of each essential oil until the liniment is effective for you. In most cases, the "less is more" principle is the best one to follow. However, because everyone is different, it's sometimes necessary to modify a remedy to make it work for some individuals.

Herbal and Aromatherapy Back Liniment

YIELD: ABOUT 3 OUNCES

3 ounces	St. John's wort tincture
12 drops	lavender essential oil
12 drops	sandalwood essential oil

Follow the method for making liniments, page 80.

APPLICATION INSTRUCTIONS: Shake well before using. Apply directly to the affected area as needed.

BACTERIAL VAGINOSIS

Bacterial vaginosis, an infection of the vagina, affects millions of women and is associated with several serious health conditions, some specific to pregnant women. For example, it has been connected with a two to three times increase in the rate of preterm labor and delivery, premature rupture of the amniotic sac, urinary tract infections, and endometritis (swelling of the endometrium).

The source of bacterial vaginosis is poorly understood despite studies of vaginal cultures. Several bacteria have been implicated in bacterial vaginosis, such as *Gardnerella vaginalis* and *Mobiluncus curtisii*; however, these species are also found in women who do not have bacterial vaginosis, making the accurate reporting of symptoms essential for diagnosis.

Topical treatment of bacterial vaginosis can be helpful. Following is a sitz bath remedy that promotes healing and alleviates discomfort.

Sitz Bath for Bacterial Vaginosis

YIELD: ENOUGH FOR 1 SITZ BATH

1 gallon	**water**
1 cup	**witch hazel** (see page 116 for how to make witch hazel)
1½ cups	**dried calendula flowers**
1½ cups	**dried yarrow flowers**
1 or 2 drops	**tea tree essential oil**

Follow the method for making a sitz bath, page 87.

USAGE INSTRUCTIONS: Soak the vaginal area for about 20 minutes.

CARPAL TUNNEL SYNDROME

Did you know that when you are pregnant you can be more likely to develop carpal tunnel syndrome? This can be caused by increased fluid retention, which puts pressure on the median nerve. Carpal tunnel syndrome that occurs during pregnancy often resolves on its own after the pregnancy is over.

A common and effective way to alleviate discomfort and provide support to the wrist is to wear a sturdy wrist stabilizer, which can be purchased at most pharmacies. Before shopping for one, ask your doctor what type they recommend.

Herbal Remedies for Carpal Tunnel

Carpal tunnel syndrome can be relieved by using topical treatments, over-the-counter products, or drinking herbal teas or other beverages that work as gentle diuretics to help your body remove excess fluid. You won't have to go very far to find most of the following remedies:

ARNICA CREAM OR GEL. Although arnica essential oil is not safe to use during pregnancy, creams or gels that are made from arnica flowers can be used. They can be applied to the wrist, forearm, and other sore areas in the arms and shoulders. An infused oil (see page 81) made with arnica flowers can be applied the same way.

CAYENNE OINTMENT. You can find cayenne ointment at most drug stores, at Asian markets, and in the pharmacy section of big-box stores and grocery stores. It can be applied to the wrist area.

GREEN TEA. Drinking bona fide green tea—not green-tea beverages—has been found to be useful in lessening carpal tunnel pain. Follow the method for making teas as infusions, page 81.

LEMON WATER. Lemon water, made with freshly squeezed lemon juice, is also a mild diuretic, so sipping on this all day can alleviate excess fluid buildup, potentially relieving pressure on the wrist. Squeeze the juice of ½ lemon into 8 ounces of water and drink.

MARSHMALLOW ROOT TEA. Useful for soothing inflamed tissues, marshmallow root can be made into a tea. Follow the method for making teas as infusions, page 81, and drink 1 to 3 cups per day.

NETTLE TEA. Another gentle diuretic, nettle tea can also relieve pressure and swelling. Follow the method for making teas as infusions, page 81, using dried nettles.

PINEAPPLE. Pineapple contains bromelain, an enzyme that decreases inflammation, swelling, and pain. It is often suggested for carpal tunnel syndrome. Simply eating pineapple can reduce the effects of carpal tunnel syndrome. Alternatively, take a bromelain supplement; ask your care provider to suggest a dosage.

ST. JOHN'S WORT. Either use St. John's wort infused oil (see the method for making infused oils, page 81), which you can apply to your wrists and arms as needed, or make a strong tea (see the method for making teas as infusions, page 81), which you can use to make a cold compress to apply to your wrist. You can even just make a cup of St. John's wort tea, let it cool, and wet a washcloth and apply the cloth to your wrist.

If the compress or cloth is hot, the heat will worsen carpal tunnel pain because it causes the tissues in the narrow passageway to swell.

TURMERIC ROOT INFUSED OIL. You can buy or make this infused oil (see the method for making infused oils, page 81). Simply apply the infused oil to the affected wrist. Alternatively, make a strong turmeric tea, let it cool, and use it to make a cold compress to apply to your wrist (see the method for making compresses, page 85).

CONSTIPATION

If you have fewer than three bowel movements in a week and the stools are hard to pass, you are experiencing constipation. Increased levels of estrogen and progesterone during pregnancy contribute to this problem. The first step in preventing constipation is to drink plenty of water, eat a lot of fresh vegetables, and consume a variety of fresh fruits, such as apricots, peaches, pears, and plums.

Taking laxative pills for constipation while you're pregnant is not recommended because they can cause uterine contractions and dehydration. Using mineral oil, a standard constipation therapy, also is not advised because it can decrease nutrient absorption.

Some helpful herbs that are used in treating constipation are aniseeds, chamomile, dried nettles, lemon balm leaves, and spearmint. Following are some simple herbal remedies:

DANDELION LEAVES. Fresh dandelion leaves can be eaten raw in a salad or steamed; dried dandelion leaves can be used to make tea. Follow the method for making teas as infusions, page 81.

FENUGREEK SEED TEA. Fenugreek seed tea bags can be purchased or the tea can be made from fenugreek seeds. To make the tea, combine 1 teaspoon of crushed fenugreek seeds with 1 cup of boiling water and let steep for 3 to 5 minutes. You may find 1 cup of the tea effective, but if necessary, drink 2 to 3 cups per day.

MARSHMALLOW ROOT TEA. Useful for soothing inflamed tissue, marshmallow root can be made into a tea. Follow the method for making teas as infusions, page 81, and drink 2 cups per day.

SENNA LEAVES. Senna is a strong laxative, and the herb should not be used by breastfeeding mothers. During pregnancy, use senna leaves with care and only if other remedies do not work. Senna leaves can cause intestinal cramping and should not be taken in high doses or for long periods of time. If used, senna leaves should always be part of a blend of herbs (see Herbal Laxative Tea, below) and not used alone. You can also buy a senna-based laxative in most drugstores.

If diet changes and herbal remedies do not resolve your constipation, talk to your midwife or doctor about safe, gentle, and effective pharmaceutical or herbal options that are stronger.

Herbal Laxative Tea

YIELD: 6½ TEASPOONS DRIED TEA

2 teaspoons	**chamomile flowers**
2 teaspoons	**lemon balm leaves**
2 teaspoons	**senna leaves**
½ teaspoon	**aniseeds**

Follow the method for making herbal teas as infusions, page 81. Let steep for 20 minutes.

DOSAGE INSTRUCTIONS: Drink 1 cup.

DRY SKIN

There are many causes of dry skin, including diet and weather. During pregnancy, dry skin can be caused by hormonal fluctuations. In addition, some pregnant women are more sensitive to any chemical that may touch their skin, such as those in soaps, laundry detergents, or scented products. Sometimes a topical yeast infection can cause dry skin and itching in such areas as the armpits, feet, skin folds, and vagina.

Dietary changes that can help combat dry skin include consuming fatty fruits and oils, such as avocados, coconut oil, olive oil, pumpkin seed oil, and sesame oil. The oils can be drizzled on popcorn, salads, and vegetables and added to smoothies. Also be sure to eat plenty of vibrantly colored fruits and vegetables, making them part of every meal. (Ideally, your plate should be loaded with vegetables or fruit whenever you make yourself a meal.) Niacin-rich foods, such as eggs and nuts, are also beneficial.

Salves offer great protection for dry skin, serving as a barrier from the environment. Infused oils, massage oils, and bath "teas" can also be helpful. Some great nourishing herbs for dry skin are aloe vera, calendula, chickweed, comfrey, German chamomile, and plantain. Chickweed, for example, can be made into a wonderful massage oil or salve. Some essential oils that are great for treating dry skin and can be added to baths, massage oils, and salves are lavender, rose hip seed oil, and sandalwood.

Infused Oil for Dry Skin

YIELD: VARIABLE

1 part	**dried calendula flowers**
1 part	**dried comfrey leaves**
1 part	**dried plantain leaves**
1 part	**dried St. John's wort**

Follow the method for making infused oils, page 81.

APPLICATION INSTRUCTIONS: Shake well before using. Apply to dry skin as needed.

Dry Skin Bath Tea

YIELD: ENOUGH FOR 1 BATH

3 cups	**dried German chamomile flowers**
1 cup	**dried calendula flowers**
1 cup	**fresh chickweed** (see note)
1 tablespoon	**coconut oil**

Put the chamomile, calendula, and chickweed in a very large bowl. Fill a kettle with water and bring to a boil over high heat. Pour over the herbs and let steep while you boil another kettle of water. Add the water and let steep for 20 minutes. Pour through a large fine-mesh strainer or colander into another bowl and cover the herbs again with boiling water until you have at least 1 gallon of bath tea. Add the coconut oil and stir to dissolve.

USAGE INSTRUCTIONS: Draw a bath and add the bath tea.

NOTE: Use only fresh chickweed for this remedy; if none is available, omit.

EXCESSIVE VOMITING (HYPEREMESIS GRAVIDARUM)

Although 70 to 80 percent of pregnant women experience morning sickness, some women suffer from the less common but much more serious hyperemesis gravidarum, which involves excessive vomiting, severe nausea, weight loss, dehydration, and imbalance. Not to be dismissed as "just morning sickness," hyperemesis gravidarum can require hospitalization and IV therapy to replace fluids.

There are important distinctions between morning sickness and hyperemesis gravidarum. Morning sickness involves nausea accompanied by some vomiting; in general, the nausea eases about twelve weeks into pregnancy. When you have morning sickness, you're able to keep down some food and unlikely to become seriously dehydrated. In contrast, hyperemesis gravidarum is characterized by severe and potentially violent vomiting that prevents you from keeping down anything, leading to dehydration. In addition, the nausea does not subside as the pregnancy progresses.

Following are the signs and symptoms of hyperemesis gravidarum:

- severe vomiting and nausea
- decreased urinary output and less urge to go
- dehydration (can be linked to headaches, confusion, and fainting)
- drastic, rapid weight loss (5 percent or more of prepregnancy weight)
- extreme fatigue
- jaundice (yellowish staining of the skin and the whites of the eyes)
- loss of elasticity in skin (due to dehydration)
- low blood pressure
- no desire for food
- rapid heart rate
- secondary depression, anxiety, or both

In general, hyperemesis gravidarum occurs more often in women who are pregnant for the first time, are underweight or severely overweight, have gastroesophageal reflux disease, have low blood pressure, or have anxiety disorders. I have most often seen it in women who are slightly underweight and experiencing their first pregnancy.

Because dehydration and electrolyte imbalance are big concerns, herbal remedies such as broths and teas can be essential in helping you maintain sufficient body fluids; however, IV therapy may be required in some cases. Other remedies are effective in reducing nausea:

CANNABIS. If medical marijuana is legal where you live, talk to your doctor about using a tincture or other form to combat nausea.

GINGER. Whether you make ginger tea as an infusion or use ginger chews or pastilles, ginger can prevent nausea. To make a tea, use 1 slice of fresh ginger per 1 cup of boiling water (see method, page 81). Alternatively, use a ginger tea bag.

PEACH LEAF TEA. Available loose or in tea bags, peach leaf tea can help relieve nausea.

Antinausea Tea Blend 1

YIELD: 1½ CUPS DRIED TEA

½ cup	**dried lemon balm leaves**
½ cup	**dried nettle leaves**
½ cup	**dried peppermint leaves**

Follow the method for making herbal teas as infusions, page 81.

DOSAGE INSTRUCTIONS: Sip throughout the day to prevent nausea.

Antinausea Tea Blend 2

YIELD: 4 CUPS PREPARED TEA

4 cups	**water**
1 tablespoon	**chopped fresh orange peel**
1 teaspoon	**chopped fresh ginger**
1 teaspoon	**dried lemon balm leaves**

Pour the water into a medium saucepan over high heat and bring to a boil. Stir in the orange peel, ginger, and lemon balm. Decrease the heat to low and let simmer for 5 minutes. Remove from the heat and let steep, covered, for 20 minutes.

DOSAGE INSTRUCTIONS: Drink 1 cup 2 or 3 times per day.

Electrolyte Formula

YIELD: 4¼ CUPS

1 quart	**coconut water**
¼ cup	**brewed nettle or lemon balm leaf tea**
1 tablespoon	**grade B maple syrup or molasses**
¼ teaspoon	**calcium-magnesium powder**
¼ teaspoon	**sea salt** (see note)

Put all the ingredients in a blender and process for 1 minute. Store in a container in the refrigerator.

DOSAGE INSTRUCTIONS: Drink 2 to 3 cups per day. If advised by a doctor or midwife, you may increase this to 5 to 6 cups. You can also make this formula into popsicles or add it to freshly made juice.

NOTE: Celtic, fleur de sel, and Himalayan are all good choices when buying sea salt.

Super Nutrition Broth

8 cups	**water**
1	**butternut or acorn squash, chopped**
2 cups	**chopped kale or collard greens**
2 cups	**coarsely chopped fresh young stinging nettles, or ¾ cup dried nettles**
6 stalks	**celery**
4	**carrots, halved**
1	**onion, halved**
4 to 6 slices	(½ inch thick) **dried reishi mushrooms**
1 slice	(½ inch thick) **fresh ginger**
	Sea salt

Put the water, squash, kale, nettles, celery, carrots, onion, mushrooms, and ginger in a large stockpot and bring to a simmer over medium heat. Decrease the heat to low, cover, and cook for 3 hours. If necessary, add additional water to keep the vegetables well covered. Strain the liquid into another pot. Season with salt to taste.

USAGE INSTRUCTIONS: Sip throughout the day.

NOTE: To store, pour into an ice-cube tray and freeze. Heat in small amounts as needed.

FAINTING AND DIZZINESS

Fainting and dizziness can occur during pregnancy, putting the mother at risk for falling. One simple way to avoid these problems is to remain reasonably active so your circulation remains strong. Body movement, such as belly dancing, stretching, and yoga (even chair yoga), will help you feel steadier on your feet.

If you experience dizziness accompanied by abdominal pain or vaginal bleeding, contact your care provider immediately. These could be signs of serious complications, including ectopic pregnancy, a low-lying placenta, or placental abruption (separation of the placenta from the uterus). In addition, contact your care provider if you are frequently dizzy or experience dizziness combined with blurred vision, headaches, or palpitations. These could be symptoms of severe anemia or other unwanted conditions that could affect your pregnancy. Because most fainting during pregnancy is caused by anemia, dehydration, and nausea, Nutritional Tea (see remedy, page 106) is wonderful for prevention.

Inhalations for Dizziness

YIELD: MULTIPLE USES

10 drops	**peppermint essential oil**
1	**handkerchief or paper towel**
1	**ziplock bag**

Put the essential oil on the handkerchief and store it in a sealed ziplock bag.

USAGE INSTRUCTIONS: Inhale the bag contents when feeling dizzy or faint.

VARIATION: Instead of putting the essential oil on a handkerchief, add it to a small amount of rock salt and store in a small, lidded container. Seal tightly.

Smelling Salts

YIELD: ABOUT ½ CUP; ENOUGH FOR SEVERAL SMALL CONTAINERS

½ cup	**rock salt**
50 drops	**eucalyptus essential oil**

Put the rock salt in a small bowl. Add the essential oil. Stir until well combined. Divide into small containers (see note).

USAGE INSTRUCTIONS: Inhale the contents of the container when feeling faint.

NOTE: Any tightly sealed small jar can be used for storing smelling salts. If you'd like the genuine article, look for antique containers designed especially for carrying smelling salts.

Nutritional Tea

YIELD: 2¼ CUPS DRIED TEA

1 cup	**dried lemon balm leaves**
1 cup	**dried nettles**
¼ cup	**diced seeded rose hips**

Follow the method for making herbal teas as infusions, page 81. Let steep for 20 minutes.

DOSAGE INSTRUCTIONS: Drink 2 to 3 cups per day.

FATIGUE

Fatigue is common early on during pregnancy, before twenty weeks. This can be attributed to a number of factors, including anemia, low blood pressure and blood sugar levels, and hormonal changes. In particular, rising levels of progesterone can cause sleepiness during early pregnancy. Some herbs that can help alleviate fatigue are alfalfa, nettles, and rose hips.

Proper nutrition is also important, so be sure to eat high-quality protein, fresh fruits and vegetables, and whole grains. Eating frequent snacks or small meals throughout the day can also help to combat fatigue. Drink plenty of water and stay away from sweets and excess caffeine. When you can, take a brisk walk or nap.

Fatigue Tea

YIELD: 1¼ CUPS DRIED TEA

½ cup	**dried hibiscus flowers**
½ cup	**dried milky oats**
¼ cup	**dried peppermint leaves**

Follow the method for making herbal teas as infusions, page 81.

DOSAGE INSTRUCTIONS: Drink 2 to 3 cups per day.

GESTATIONAL DIABETES

Gestational diabetes refers to diabetes that a woman develops during pregnancy; it occurs in women who are not already diabetic. Diabetes arises when the body does not produce or appropriately use insulin, a hormone necessary to convert sugar, starches, and other foods into energy. According to the National Institutes of Health, gestational diabetes occurs in about 5 percent of all pregnancies in the United States, resulting in about 200,000 cases a year.

Although the issues associated with this form of diabetes cease after the mother gives birth, according to the US Centers for Disease Control, about half the women with gestational diabetes will also have type 2 diabetes later in life. Therefore, the presence of gestational diabetes can indicate the need to make lifestyle changes for prevention's sake.

Gestational diabetes doesn't always have many noticeable symptoms, and women may overlook the signs. Commonly, it is diagnosed during prenatal checkups. Some indicators of gestational diabetes follow:

- blurred vision
- excessive thirst
- increased urination
- infections
- nausea and vomiting

Certain factors make gestational diabetes more likely to occur in some women. For example, obesity is one risk factor, although gestational diabetes is now frequently being diagnosed in women who aren't overweight. In addition, women older than age thirty are more likely to have gestational diabetes. Other risk factors include the following:

- elevated blood pressure
- gestational diabetes during a previous pregnancy
- history of diabetes in the family

A number of herbal remedies can be useful if you have gestational diabetes. Following are a few suggestions:

BITTER MELON. A popular food in Asia, bitter melon is a member of the squash family and can be included like any other vegetable in curries, soups, and stir-fries. Bitter melon can also be used to make a tea, which you can have upon rising in the morning. **Caution:** Use only under supervision, as bitter melon can cause uterine contractions (see pages 51 to 52).

CINNAMON. Cinnamon is known for maintaining a healthy balance of blood sugar. Using as little as one-half teaspoon per day can be effective. Use a high-quality cinnamon, stirring it into tea or a smoothie or sprinkling it on fruits, toast, or vegetables.

FENUGREEK SEEDS. Easy to make into tea (see Fenugreek Seed Tea, page 100), this common spice-drawer ingredient is also delicious on savory foods. Incorporate more fenugreek into your diet by keeping some in a pepper grinder and using it as a seasoning.

GURMAR. Sold in capsule form, this herb can be an effective treatment for gestational diabetes, but should be used only under the supervision of a doctor or midwife. Take one or two capsules after meals.

GROUP B STREPTOCOCCUS

Group B streptococcus, commonly referred to as group B strep, is a species of bacteria that many people have in their intestinal tracts. The bacteria may also occupy, or colonize in, the vagina and rectum, so it can be passed on to a baby during labor and birth. Colonization in the rectum and vagina is more likely to occur when there is improper wiping after defecation (never wipe from back to front) or as a result of sexual intercourse (especially when anal sex immediately precedes vaginal sex).

Infection with group B strep poses risks for both mother and baby. The mother may miscarry or experience intra-amniotic infection. She may also be subject to sepsis, an infection in the blood. If infected with group B strep, the baby can also be at risk for sepsis, meningitis, or pneumonia. Five percent of babies born with these conditions don't survive. Preterm infants have a lower survival rate than full-term babies, and those who survive are at higher risk for having long-term side effects. Surviving babies, particularly those with meningitis, can have serious health problems, such as cerebral palsy, developmental disabilities, and hearing or vision loss.

Because it may not be possible to adequately predict whether a mother is infected before delivery, taking steps during pregnancy to eradicate or reduce infection is advisable. Many natural treatments are effective in decreasing colonization and the potential for passing it along to the baby. Following are several effective remedies to try:

ACIDOPHILUS CAPSULES. Take 6 to 8 capsules per day. In addition, you can open a capsule and sprinkle the contents directly on the vagina.

ECHINACEA TINCTURE. Use echinacea tincture during the last two weeks of pregnancy, from thirty-nine weeks on. Take 2 millimeters, 3 times per day.

GARLIC IN THE DIET. Eat 3 to 4 raw cloves of garlic daily. Crush the garlic slightly before eating it, and consume it with some citrus fruit because garlic is most effective when paired with vitamin C.

GARLIC SUPPOSITORIES. Insert 1 to 2 bruised and peeled garlic cloves into the vagina per day; to bruise a clove, put an unpeeled clove on a clean counter and roll it under your palm. Alternatively, insert the garlic into the vagina every other night, or every three nights, prior to bedtime. Continue until delivery.

LAVENDER OR TEA TREE ESSENTIAL OIL BATHS. Given their antibacterial properties, these essential oils provide not only a relaxing but also a healing bath. In a full bath, add 10 drops of lavender or tea tree essential oil, either alone or in combination.

NASTURTIUM BLOSSOMS. Enjoy the peppery flavor of these edible flowers, which are sometimes compared to those of radishes, in salads or stirred into soups.

PROBIOTICS. Open a probiotic capsule and sprinkle the contents directly on the vagina. Alternatively, insert a probiotic capsule into the vagina before going to sleep and allow it to dissolve in the vagina overnight.

REISHI TEA. The reishi mushroom is known for its healing properties. You can make reishi tea using fresh mushrooms or buy the dried form in easy-to-use tea bags, which are available at most natural food stores. Drink the tea throughout pregnancy.

SHIITAKE MUSHROOMS. Like all mushrooms, shiitake mushrooms are considered both an herb and a food. They contain antiviral and antibacterial agents and are known to boost the immune system.

VITAMIN C-RICH HERBS. Include nourishing herbs, such as coriander, hibiscus, and rose hips, in your diet.

YOGURT AND KEFIR. Fermented dairy products that contain probiotics, such as yogurt and kefir, are easy to find in supermarkets. Consume them as is or stir healthful herbs into these products to make dips and sauces. Some traditional choices include cilantro, garlic, and mint.

Tampon Remedy 1 for Group B Strep

YIELD: 4 TAMPONS

4 cups	**water**
8 tablespoons	**fresh lavender**
8 tablespoons	**fresh rosemary**
1 drop	**rosemary essential oil**
4	**tampons**

Pour the water into a medium saucepan over high heat and bring to a boil. Fill a quart jar with the lavender and rosemary and cover with the boiling water. Let cool. Stir in the rosemary essential oil. Immerse the tampons in the liquid. Let soak for 1 hour.

USAGE INSTRUCTIONS: Insert one of the tampons into the vagina and keep it there for 3 hours. Remove the tampon. Wait 1 hour and put in the second tampon. Store the third and fourth tampons in the container in the refrigerator, and follow the same regimen the next day.

NOTE: Use any leftover liquid to make vaginal and rectal wipes. Fold 8 to 10 paper towels and put them in a square plastic container. Cover with the liquid. Use the towels to wipe after having a bowel movement. Keep unused towels covered and stored in the refrigerator for no more than 4 days.

Tampon Remedy 2 for Group B Strep

1 cup	**chickweed tea**
2 tablespoons	**thyme tincture**
2 tablespoons	**usnea tincture**
3 drops	**lavender essential oil**
4	**tampons**

Put the chickweed tea, thyme tincture, usnea tincture, and lavender essential oil in a quart jar. Stir to combine. Immerse the tampons in the liquid. Let soak for 1 hour.

USAGE INSTRUCTIONS: Use as described for Tampon Remedy 1.

Suppository for Group B Strep

1 cup	**cocoa butter or shea butter**
½ cup	**coconut oil**
2 tablespoons	**calendula-infused oil**
1 tablespoon	**plantain-infused oil**
½ teaspoon	**lavender essential oil**
½ teaspoon	**tea tree essential oil**
¼ teaspoon	**sandalwood essential oil**
4 tablespoons	**powdered plantain leaves**
2 tablespoons	**goldenseal root powder**
¼ teaspoon	**powdered dried thyme**

Put the cocoa butter and coconut oil in a small saucepan over low heat until melted. Remove from the heat. Stir in both the calendula- and plantain-infused oils. Add the lavender, tea tree, and sandalwood essential oils and the plantain leaves, goldenseal, and thyme. Stir until well combined. Pour into an ice-cube tray with 18 compartments and freeze until firm. Remove from the freezer and store in the refrigerator.

USAGE INSTRUCTIONS: Slice in half lengthwise to use. Insert 1 suppository into the vagina for 7 nights; repeat as needed.

NOTE: The suppository will melt throughout the night. To protect the bedding, you may want to wear a panty shield or sleep with a towel beneath you.

Immune-Boosting Tincture

·YIELD: VARIABLE

1 part	**echinacea root**
1 part	**dried nettles**
1 part	**dried peppermint leaves**
½ part	**dried rose hips**

Follow the method for making tinctures, page 83.

DOSAGE INSTRUCTIONS: Take 20 drops orally, 2 times per day for 10 days. Do not use the tincture for 2 days, then repeat the dosage as often as you like until the onset of labor.

HEADACHE

Headaches can occur during pregnancy for many reasons, including exhaustion, fatigue, hormonal swings, hunger, low blood sugar, and stress. To prevent headaches, drink plenty of water, strive for proper nutrition, exercise, and get enough rest. Frequently eating small meals can also help.

Contact your care provider if you experience headaches that are different from normal. In addition, seek medical care if you have headaches that are accompanied by any of the following symptoms: blurry, spotty, or starry vision; pain in the upper right abdomen; sudden weight gain; or swelling of the hands and face.

Some simple remedies that can be helpful in treating headaches include cold or warm compresses, head massage, and a warm bath or shower. Sometimes headaches are caused by congestion; a steam inhalation (see page 6) containing essential oils, such as lavender or tea tree, can clear congestion and alleviate this type of headache. Steam inhalation can also be helpful for stress and exhaustion headaches. To get even more benefit, when the water has cooled, use it to make a compress: soak a hand towel in the liquid, wring out the towel so it's damp but not dripping, and wrap it around your head. If you carry stress in the neck, wrap a compress, either cool or warm, around the neck.

Aromatherapy can also be beneficial for headaches. Some great essential oils to use are lavender, lemon, peppermint, spearmint, sweet orange, and tea tree.

As is the case for so many ailments, a cup of hot tea can do wonders for a headache. One simple remedy is to prepare a cup of caffeinated black tea and stir in ¼ teaspoon of cinnamon. In addition to easing headache pain, cinnamon also regulates blood sugar, which can be helpful in alleviating headaches related to hunger. The following tea remedies are also excellent for headaches.

Headache Tea for Pregnancy

YIELD: 2 CUPS DRIED TEA

½ cup	**dried lemon balm leaves**
½ cup	**dried nettles**
½ cup	**dried rose hips**
½ cup	**dried spearmint leaves**

Follow the method for making herbal teas as infusions, page 81. Use 1 tablespoon of tea per 2 cups of water. Let steep for 20 to 30 minutes.

DOSAGE INSTRUCTIONS: Drink 2 to 3 times per day.

Headache Chai

YIELD: 3 CUPS PREPARED TEA

3 cups	**water**
1	**cinnamon stick**
1 (1-inch) piece	**ginger root, peeled and thinly sliced**
6	**whole green cardamom pods**
4	**whole black peppercorns**
4	**whole cloves**
2	**black tea bags, or 1 tablespoon loose black tea**
1 cup	**milk** (optional)
1 to 2 tablespoons	**maple syrup, agave nectar, sugar, or other sweetener** (optional)

Put the water, cinnamon, ginger, cardamom, peppercorns, cloves, and tea in a medium saucepan over high heat and bring to a boil. Decrease the heat to low, partially cover, and simmer for 20 minutes. Remove from the heat. Pour into a teapot and stir in the milk and maple syrup if desired.

DOSAGE INSTRUCTIONS: Drink 2 to 3 cups per day.

VARIATION: If you prefer less caffeine, use green tea instead of black tea.

HEARTBURN

Heartburn is a sore, burning feeling in the chest, throat, or both. It occurs when stomach acid rises up into the esophagus, which is the tube that carries food from the mouth to the stomach. Uncomfortable and annoying, heartburn is common during pregnancy.

Some actions that contribute to indigestion and heartburn are over-eating, eating too fast, swallowing air, and improper chewing. Mindful chewing is one way to prevent heartburn. Try chewing each mouthful twenty times. In addition, don't drink a lot while eating; instead, drink before or after your meal.

If heartburn is a problem for you, there are both aromatherapy and herbal remedies that can help. For example, citrus essential oils are especially effective in relieving heartburn. Following are some simple but effective herbal remedies:

ANISE, DILL, AND FENNEL SEEDS. Add these herbs to recipes, use them to make a decoction (see page 81), or use them alone or combined to make a tea by adding 1 teaspoon of seeds to 1 cup of boiling water.

FENNEL SEEDS. Chew a few seeds when you feel heartburn coming on.

HERBAL TEA. Dried chamomile flowers, dried dandelion leaves, and ginger can be used, either separately or in combination, to make teas that can help to relieve heartburn. Follow the method for making teas as infusions, page 81, using 1 teaspoon of dried tea per 1 cup of boiling water. One caution: Because dandelion tea can be a strong diuretic, it's not recommended if you have gestational diabetes or take prescription medicine for high blood pressure.

SLIPPERY ELM LOZENGES. Sucking on these lozenges, which can be found at natural food stores, lubricates and coats the esophagus, helping to relieve heartburn discomfort. You can safely use 8 to 12 lozenges per day.

Blended Oil for Heartburn

YIELD: ABOUT 6 OUNCES

6 ounces	**vegetable oil**
10 drops	**lemon essential oil**
10 drops	**mandarin essential oil**
10 drops	**sweet orange essential oil**

Follow the method for making blended oils, page 79.

APPLICATION INSTRUCTIONS: Massage a little of this oil into your chest. Alternatively, put some on a tissue and smell it when you feel heartburn coming on.

NOTE: If the oil is not strong enough, add more essential oil, 2 drops at a time, until an effective strength is achieved.

Heartburn Tea

YIELD: 3 CUPS DRIED TEA

1 cup	**dried raspberry leaves**
½ cup	**dried chamomile flowers**
½ cup	**dried lemon balm leaves**
½ cup	**marshmallow root**
½ cup	**dried spearmint leaves**

Follow the method for making herbal teas as infusions, page 81.

DOSAGE INSTRUCTIONS: Drink 1 cup after eating a meal or upon the onset of heartburn.

HEMORRHOIDS

Hemorrhoids are swollen veins in the anal canal. For some women, hemorrhoids can occur during the last six months of pregnancy, when an increased load is put on the blood vessels in the pelvic area. Hemorrhoids are a fairly common problem and can be painful and irritating; generally, however, they are not serious and can often be treated with herbal remedies. Helpful herbs are chickweed, shepherd's purse, spearmint, and witch hazel (see Witch Hazel Extract, page 116). Following are some useful topical treatments made from herbs:

COMPRESSES. Teas, extracts, or tinctures made from the following herbs can be used to make cold compresses (see method, page 85): parsley, plantain leaves, sage, shepherd's purse, St. John's wort, and witch hazel. Apply to the affected area.

OINTMENTS. Over-the-counter ointments or homemade salves (see method, page 85) made from the following herbs can provide relief from hemorrhoids: comfrey, peony root, witch hazel, and yarrow. Apply to the affected area.

PANTY LINERS. To treat external hemorrhoids, soak a panty liner or cloth with one or two of the following teas (see method, page 81) or tinctures (see method, page 83): parsley, plantain leaves, sage, shepherd's purse, St. John's wort, and witch hazel. Put the panty liner or cloth over the affected area and pull on cotton panties to hold it in place. Do this at night when you're sleeping or when you will be staying relatively still, such as when you're watching a movie or reading a book.

WITCH HAZEL WIPES. A classic treatment to soothe hemorrhoids, tears, and swelling, is to wet a soft flannel cloth with witch hazel to use as a wipe. Alternatively, make wipes by placing cotton pads from the drugstore in a small plastic container and covering them with witch hazel.

YARROW. An astringent that works to constrict hemorrhoids, yarrow is beneficial when used as a compress (see method, page 85) or in a sitz bath (see method, page 87). For the best results, use it in combination with comfrey and witch hazel.

Witch Hazel Extract

YIELD: ABOUT 2 CUPS

1 cup	**dried witch hazel leaves**
1 cup	**80-proof vodka or rum**
1 cup	**water**
5 to 10 drops	**cypress essential oil** (optional)

Put the witch hazel in a jar and cover with the vodka and water. Put the lid on the jar and close tightly. Let steep for 4 weeks. Strain and pour into a clean bottle. Add the cypress essential oil if desired. Put the cap on the bottle and close tightly.

Hemorrhoid Salve

YIELD: 2 CUPS

1 cup	**shredded beeswax** (see note)
½ cup	**St. John's wort infused oil**
¼ cup	**calendula-infused oil**
¼ cup	**horse chestnut extract**

Follow the method for making salves, page 80.

APPLICATION INSTRUCTIONS: Apply to the affected area as needed.

NOTE: Candelilla wax or coconut oil can be used in place of beeswax.

Hemorrhoid Ointment

YIELD: 1½ CUPS

¼ cup	**comfrey leaf infused oil**
¼ cup	**parsley-infused oil**
¼ cup	**St. John's wort infused oil**
¼ cup	**yarrow-infused oil** (see note)
½ to ¾ ounce	**shredded beeswax**

Put the infused oils in a medium saucepan over very low heat. Slowly stir in the beeswax until it melts. Store in a widemouthed container that can be closed securely.

APPLICATION INSTRUCTIONS: Apply to the affected area as needed.

NOTE: See the method for making infused oils, page 81. This ointment is runnier and softer than a salve. Be sure to use yarrow-infused oil and not yarrow essential oil, which should not be used during pregnancy.

HERPES

Herpes in pregnancy can cause multiple complications. For example, an active herpes outbreak may be a justifiable reason for a C-section, for the health of both the mother and the baby. The good news is that some herbs can be quite effective in preventing an outbreak. These include nervines, such as lemon balm and passionflower, and antivirals, such as black walnut and garlic.

I have known many women who have prevented a herpes outbreak around delivery time simply by using lemon balm tea topically and taking it internally. Lemon balm not only supports the nervous system but also acts as an antiviral. As an antiviral, lemon balm can temporarily suppress an outbreak; as a nervine, it lessens stress levels that are outbreak triggers for some women. In addition to a healing tea, lemon balm can be made into a compress, an infused oil, or an ointment. Any of these can be used topically if you feel what are described as the "tingles" of a herpes outbreak coming on.

HYPERTENSION

Hypertension, or high blood pressure, can occur during pregnancy. In part, it can be prevented by exercise and controlled by diet. For example, eating a lot of cucumber is known to lower blood pressure, as is eating garlic, fresh stinging nettles, and onions. If you prefer, you can use garlic tablets instead of eating fresh garlic.

After the first trimester, several herbal teas can help control high blood pressure. Drinking a cup of hops tea every night can help you sleep and relax. Passionflower tea can do the same. In addition, dried nettles and raspberry leaves are good choices. In fact, both are featured in most ready-made pregnancy teas because they are effective in controlling blood pressure. Preeclampsia (see page 122) is a condition that causes pregnant women to develop very high blood pressure. More serious than standard hypertension, preeclampsia requires medical supervision.

INSOMNIA

Sleep can be difficult to come by during pregnancy. Having a comfortable sleeping position is essential, and props such as body pillows or specially shaped neck pillows have made it easier for many women to get through the night. Insomnia during pregnancy has many causes beyond discomfort, including heartburn, hormonal changes, stress, and the frequent need to urinate during the night. Aromatherapy and herbal remedies offer a variety of solutions.

Herbs that can lull you into dreamland include lavender, lemon balm, passionflower, skullcap, rooibos, and rose hips. These are incorporated in some of the following remedies:

DRIED LAVENDER. The scent of dried lavender flowers in or around your bed can help lull you to sleep. Either put a few sprigs under the fitted sheet so that the scent is released as you move in your sleep or put a bouquet of dried lavender near your bed.

HERBAL TEA. Teas made from dried chamomile flowers, dried lavender flowers, or dried lemon balm leaves, used singly or in combination, can promote sleep. Follow the method for making teas as infusions, page 81, using 1 teaspoon of dried tea per 1 cup of water. Alternatively, use a sleep-inducing tea from the grocery store or natural food store. Drink the tea right before bedtime.

LAVENDER ESSENTIAL OIL BATH. A bath before bedtime can be relaxing and prepare you for restful sleep. Draw a warm bath and add a few drops of lavender essential oil.

SACHET. A sachet is a small cloth bag, usually between five and seven inches wide, full of fragrant herbs. Make a sachet containing cedar shavings, dried lavender flowers, dried orange peel, and dried rose petals. Hang it on the bed or place it under the pillow.

Nourishing Insomnia Tea

YIELD: 1½ CUPS DRIED TEA

½ cup **dried lemon balm leaves**

½ cup **dried raspberry leaves**

½ cup **skullcap leaves** (see note)

Follow the method for making herbal teas as infusions, page 81.

DOSAGE INSTRUCTIONS: Drink 1 cup before bedtime.

NOTE: Use skullcap (see page 65) with caution during pregnancy; use only limited amounts under supervision.

Sleeping Salve

YIELD: 2 CUPS

2 cups **carrier oil** (see box, page 14)

3 tablespoons **grated beeswax**

10 drops **lavender essential oil**

10 drops **sandalwood essential oil**

Follow the method for making salves, page 80.

APPLICATION INSTRUCTIONS: Apply the salve to your chest, bottoms of your feet, or temples to help facilitate sleep.

NOTE: Candelilla wax or coconut oil can be used in place of beeswax.

LEG CRAMPS

During pregnancy, legs cramps can range from mild to severe. They can manifest as moderate cramping and aching pain or as radiating, painful spasms in the calves. This happens especially at night, when fluid accumulates and fatigue sets in. In general, leg cramps are more likely to occur when pregnancy weight gain increases.

Some simple movements can help to relieve and prevent cramping. When leg cramps begin, straighten your leg, gently flexing your toes toward your nose. This will ease the spasm and help the pain to go away. Don't flex your toes downward, as this will make the cramp worse. While you're relaxing in the evening, circle your ankles slowly in one direction and then in the other to prevent spasms.

Another way to avoid leg cramps is to eat foods rich in magnesium and potassium. Magnesium is abundant in many common foods, including broccoli, nuts, sesame and sunflower seeds, soy milk, spinach, and tofu. Some potassium-rich foods are dried apricots, avocados, bananas, chocolate, pistachios, and pumpkin and sunflower seeds.

Some helpful herbal teas for leg cramps are dried nettle and raspberry leaf, which are good to have before bedtime; if you want to avoid getting up at night to go to the bathroom, have the tea after dinner instead. An excellent topical treatment is Leg Cramp Oil (see below), which can be applied as needed. This remedy is also soothing for back pain and varicose veins.

Leg Cramp Oil

YIELD: 2 OUNCES

2 ounces	**St. John's wort infused oil**
5 drops	**grapefruit essential oil**
5 drops	**neroli essential oil**

Follow the method for making blended oils, page 79.

APPLICATION INSTRUCTIONS: Shake well. Using a gentle upward and sweeping motion, rub into the skin on your legs before bedtime.

LOW AMNIOTIC FLUID

Mothers who are dehydrated may have low levels of amniotic fluid. In this case, the first suggestion is to increase your water intake. If this is not effective, alternative treatment, such as IV fluids, may be needed. In addition to drinking plenty of water, expecting mothers can benefit from Hydrating Tea (see below), which can increase fluid levels.

Hydrating Tea

YIELD: 1 GALLON

1 gallon	**water**
½ cup	**fresh lemon balm leaves**
½ cup	**dried rose hips**

Follow the method for making herbal teas as infusions, page 81.

DOSAGE INSTRUCTIONS: Drink 2 to 3 cups per day.

MORNING SICKNESS

Often one of the first signs of pregnancy, morning sickness is characterized by nausea and vomiting, which can strike any time of day. Morning sickness affects over 50 percent of pregnant women.

While uncomfortable, morning sickness may not be debilitating, especially if you make some lifestyle changes. It can be helpful to get regular exercise and plenty of fresh air, snack often, and avoid nausea triggers, such as greasy foods.

Essential oils and aromatherapy are particularly helpful in allaying nausea and morning sickness. For example, simply inhaling citrus, ginger, grapefruit, lemon, peppermint, or spearmint essential oils can be effective. Put a few drops on a tissue or cloth under your nose or on a washcloth on your pillow. Alternatively, put a few drops of one of these essential oils in a room diffuser to disperse them into the air.

Several herbs are effective in treating morning sickness. These include ginger, lavender, peach leaves, raspberry leaves, peppermint, and spearmint. Sip teaspoons of ginger, peppermint, or spearmint tea throughout the day. Alternatively, sip natural varieties of ginger ale or ginger beer. Try ginger candy or chews, peppermint candies, or mints to help contain nausea. You can find natural versions at herb shops or natural food stores, or you can make them yourself.

Rarely, morning sickness is so severe it's classified as hyperemesis gravidarum (see page 102), which can require hospitalization and treatment with IV fluids and antinausea medications. Contact your care provider if you experience any of the following symptoms:

- severe nausea or vomiting that does not stop
- inability to keep down fluids
- scant urine output or very dark or odorous urine
- fainting or feeling dizzy or faint upon standing
- racing heartbeat
- vomiting blood

Antinausea Tea Blend 3

YIELD: 2 CUPS DRIED TEA

1 cup **dried peach leaves**
1 cup **dried raspberry leaves**

Follow the method for making herbal teas as infusions, page 81.

DOSAGE INSTRUCTIONS: Drink 1 cup, 2 or 3 times per day, or take sips throughout the day.

Morning Sickness Tea

3 cups	**water**
2 teaspoons	**dried spearmint leaves**
1 teaspoon	**dried lemon balm leaves**
½ teaspoon	**chopped fresh ginger**
½ teaspoon	**chopped fresh orange peel**
½ teaspoon	**dried peppermint leaves**

Follow the method for making herbal teas as infusions, page 81.

DOSAGE INSTRUCTIONS: Drink 1 cup, 3 times per day, or take sips throughout the day.

PREECLAMPSIA

Also called toxemia, preeclampsia is a life-threatening illness that occurs during the later stages of pregnancy and is characterized by high blood pressure, water retention, and protein in the urine. Symptoms include headaches, visual problems, swollen ankles, nausea, and abdominal pain. If preeclampsia is left untreated, convulsions and loss of consciousness can occur, threatening the life of the mother and child.

Although preeclampsia requires emergency medical attention should it occur, herbal remedies can be used to prevent its onset or as an adjunct to conventional treatment. If you are using any herbal remedies, be sure to inform your doctor.

Routine prenatal care is vital in catching preeclampsia early, so ensure you have regular checkups. If you are diagnosed with a mild case, your doctor will advise bed rest and prescribe drugs to decrease blood pressure and correct salt and water imbalances. If you are nearing the end of your pregnancy, the decision may be made to induce birth, as symptoms rapidly improve after delivery.

A number of healthful behaviors during pregnancy can be effective in warding off the complications of preeclampsia. There are many viewpoints about this, so talk to your care provider about what might work in your situation. Following are my general recommendations:

AVOID STRESS. Decrease stress as much as possible by taking frequent naps and relaxing baths. If you have access to a pool, swimming can help regulate blood pressure.

EAT CALCIUM-RICH FOODS. In addition to low-fat dairy foods, many other options provide plentiful amounts of calcium. Dark, leafy vegetables, such as collard greens, kale, and turnip greens, are outstanding sources. Fortified foods and beverages, such as cereals, juices, and soy milk, are good choices, as are calcium-enriched breads and grain products.

EAT POTASSIUM-RICH FOODS. Food such as bananas, beets, chicory, dandelion greens, and potatoes with peels pack a potassium punch. In addition, try to add spirulina or other sea vegetables into your diet.

EAT PROTEIN-RICH FOODS. Some studies show that a diet deficient in protein may contribute to preeclampsia, so eat lean meat and fish (or vegetarian equivalents), eggs, legumes, low-fat dairy products, and whole grains. If you are a vegetarian or vegan, ensure you get sufficient protein by eating legumes, nuts, and seeds. And don't forget that all whole plant-based foods, including fruits and vegetables, also contain protein.

SLEEP. Get plenty of it.

Herbal remedies and complementary medicine can be useful in preventing or managing preeclampsia. Following are some options:

DANDELION LEAVES. Helpful in reducing swelling caused by water retention, fresh dandelion leaves can be added to salads and other dishes. Alternatively, make a decoction by putting 2 teaspoons of dandelion root and 1 cup of water in a saucepan and simmering gently for 15 minutes. Drink 3 times daily.

HERBAL TEAS. Tea blends that contain dried dandelion leaves, dried nettles, and dried raspberry leaves are good choices.

TRADITIONAL CHINESE MEDICINE. Herbs and acupuncture can be used to treat high blood pressure.

For more information about preeclampsia, visit blueribbonbaby.org.

PRURITIC URTICARIAL PAPULES AND PLAQUES OF PREGNANCY (PUPPP)

Pruritic urticarial papules and plaques of pregnancy, or PUPPP, is difficult to say and uncomfortable to endure. The term refers to an incredibly itchy and at times painful rash some women experience during pregnancy. Although the cause of the rash isn't completely understood, one potential explanation is that it's an allergic reaction to the stretching and distension of the skin. To complicate matters, women who are treated for PUPPP experience varying results. So with this issue, you may find you have to try more than one remedy.

Although most PUPPP remedies are topical, a few can be beneficial when taken internally. Following are some examples:

DRIED NETTLE TEA. Because it works as an antihistamine, dried nettle tea helps to curb the itchiness of PUPPP.

LEAFY GREENS. Herbs such as chickweed, dandelion, and stinging nettle can be eaten fresh and are especially effective when paired with other leafy greens and herbs rich in vitamin C. Dandelion tincture can be used in place of the fresh leaves.

NERVINES. Oats and plantains are foods that support the nervous system. Eating these foods or drinking teas made from them can be helpful during a PUPPP outbreak, as can using topical treatments that include oats or plantains.

A variety of household items can provide relief when applied topically, such as fresh aloe vera gel, a simple paste made from baking soda and water, cocoa butter, mint toothpaste, and rosewater. Cold showers and oat baths (see below) can also bring relief.

Topical treatments in many forms can be used to treat PUPPP. Following are some suggested remedies:

CALENDULA. Calendula, which is an anti-inflammatory and antiseptic, can be very soothing when used to treat conditions such as PUPPP, especially when the skin is broken or scratched. Various forms of calendula, including creams, ointments, and tinctures, can be used topically.

CHAMOMILE. Studies have documented that both German and Roman chamomile are effective anti-inflammatories. The herb is often made into creams or lotions or used in baths or compresses to soothe skin irritations.

OAT BATH. Oatmeal, which can be used topically or taken internally, has been a standard for relieving skin issues for over one hundred years. To make an oatmeal bath, put 1 cup of rolled oats in a food processor and process into a fine powder. Alternatively, use infant oatmeal, which is already finely milled. Draw a bath, add the oatmeal, and distribute.

Soak for 15 to 20 minutes; after leaving the tub, gently pat yourself dry. Rubbing the skin with a towel is likely to promote itching.

TOWEL COMPRESS. When it comes to topical treatments, compresses are essential for soothing itchy skin. To make a towel compress, fill a large bowl with a strong herbal tea made from calendula, chamomile, St. John's wort, strawberry leaves, witch hazel, or other soothing herbs. The tea must be cool. Soak the towel, wring it out, and drape it over the affected area for relief.

WITCH HAZEL. Witch hazel is great when used as a compress (see towel compress, above) or cream, applied as a tincture, or mixed fifty-fifty with aloe vera gel and applied directly to the skin.

PUPPP Essential Oil Blend 1

YIELD: 4 OUNCES

4 ounces	**olive oil**
10 drops	**German chamomile essential oil**
10 drops	**lavender essential oil**
10 drops	**Roman chamomile essential oil**
10 drops	**sandalwood essential oil**

Follow the method for making blended oils, page 79.

APPLICATION INSTRUCTIONS: Apply directly to the rash.

PUPPP Essential Oil Blend 2

YIELD: 4 OUNCES

2 ounces	**jojoba oil**
2 ounces	**olive oil**
14 drops	**lavender essential oil**
10 drops	**German chamomile essential oil**
10 drops	**helichrysum essential oil**
10 drops	**patchouli essential oil**
5 drops	**vitamin E oil, or 1 capsule, split open and emptied**

Follow the method for making blended oils, page 79.

APPLICATION INSTRUCTIONS: Apply directly to the rash.

PUPPP Tea

YIELD: ABOUT 2 CUPS DRIED TEA

1 cup	**dried nettles**
½ cup	**dandelion root**
½ cup	**dried milky oats**
3 tablespoons	**dried rose hips**

Follow the method for making herbal teas as infusions, page 81. Use 1 teaspoon of dried tea per 1 cup of water. Let steep for 30 minutes.

DOSAGE INSTRUCTIONS: Drink 2 to 3 cups per day.

ROUND LIGAMENT PAIN

Round ligament pain is also called pelvic girdle pain or symphysis pubic dysfunction. It occurs in the circular ligament in the pelvic region. Pregnancy and hormones can stretch the ligament, causing discomfort and sharp pains in the groin region and under the baby bump.

Most women find relief using a maternity belt, which can be purchased for as little as $15. Walks and yoga can also alleviate round ligament pain. In addition, rest can be beneficial.

Several simple herbal remedies can provide relief from the discomfort of round ligament pain. Following are some examples:

BATH WITH ESSENTIAL OILS. Draw a warm bath. Add a few drops of lavender, rose, or sandalwood essential oil. Soak for 15 to 20 minutes.

COMPRESSES. Follow the method for making warm compresses (see page 85) with herbs such as lavender, peppermint, St. John's wort, valerian, or witch hazel. Use as needed to reduce pain.

ST. JOHN'S WORT INFUSED OIL. Apply the infused oil directly to the skin as needed for pain.

Contact your care provider if you have persistent round ligament discomfort. In particular, seek help if pelvic pain is accompanied by any of the following symptoms:

- severe cramping, pain, and contractions or a contraction that doesn't end
- lower back pain, especially if new
- vaginal bleeding, spotting, or changes in vaginal discharge
- pain or burning with urination or blood in the urine

- fever or chills
- feeling faint
- nausea or vomiting

Round Ligament Massage Oil

YIELD: 1 CUP

1 cup	St. John's wort infused oil
10 drops	black pepper essential oil
10 drops	lavender essential oil

Follow the method for making blended and massage oils, page 79.

APPLICATION INSTRUCTIONS: Shake well before using. Apply to the skin in the pelvic area.

SCIATICA

Sciatica refers to pain, weakness, numbness, or tingling in the legs. These sensations originate near the buttocks and radiate outward and downward when the sciatic nerve is injured, pinched, or pressed. This can occur during pregnancy as the result of fluid retention and weight gain. Massaging the buttocks and surrounding muscles can alleviate pressure on the nerve, as can doing gentle stretches.

Treatments for sciatica can be used topically or taken internally. Following are some to try:

ARNICA. Although arnica essential oil is not safe to use during pregnancy, creams, gels, or liniments that are made from arnica flowers can be used. An infused oil (see page 81) made with arnica flowers can also be used. Apply to the affected areas.

LINIMENTS. Homemade or purchased liniments containing peppermint or valerian are good choices. Apply to the affected areas.

MASSAGE OILS. Homemade or purchased massage oils containing helichrysum or Roman chamomile can provide relief. Rub the oil into the affected areas.

ST. JOHN'S WORT. Apply St. John's wort infused oil to the affected area. In addition, drink St. John's wort herbal tea.

TURMERIC. Apply turmeric-infused oil to the affected area. In addition, to benefit from turmeric's anti-inflammatory effects, include it in foods and beverages.

Pain-Relieving Oil Blend

YIELD: 2 TABLESPOONS

2 tablespoons	**St. John's wort infused oil**
10 drops	**lavender essential oil**
10 drops	**Roman chamomile essential oil**

Follow the method for making blended oils, page 79.

APPLICATION INSTRUCTIONS: Cover one side of a square bandage, gauze pad, or washcloth with the oil and apply to the affected area. Alternatively, use as a massage oil.

VARIATION: Use St. John's wort tea instead of infused oil and make a compress. Follow the method for making compresses, page 85.

STRETCH MARKS

Stretch marks occur as the result of the abdomen's rapid expansion during pregnancy. A good strategy is to eat nourishing fats and high-quality foods that will enhance the skin's elasticity and minimize the development of stretch marks. In addition, of course, using topical remedies during this time can help limit discomfort. Following are some tried-and-true options:

COCOA BUTTER. Available in most pharmacies or online, pure cocoa butter nourishes and heals the skin. If you like, add other emollients to make Simple Stretch Mark Salve (see below). Apply to the abdomen. (Note that pure cocoa butter, like coconut oil, is solid at room temperature. Allow it to soften on the skin for a few moments before rubbing it in.)

HEALING OILS. Apply other moisturizing and healing oils, such as sesame oil or shea butter, to the abdomen. Other good choices include calendula-infused oil, plantain-infused oil, and rose petal infused oil.

Simple Stretch Mark Salve

YIELD: ABOUT ¾ CUP

½ cup	**cocoa butter**
¼ cup	**coconut oil**
2 tablespoons	**rose hip seed oil**

Follow the method for making salves, page 80.

APPLICATION INSTRUCTIONS: Apply to the abdomen regularly to keep skin soft and elastic.

VARICOSE VEINS

Varicose veins are abnormally enlarged and twisted veins near the surface of the skin. They most commonly develop in the legs and ankles but can also occur in the upper thigh and vagina. They can be quite painful and cause multiple problems during pregnancy.

Varicose veins must be treated gently. When applying topical remedies, be sure not to put direct pressure on the vein. Do not massage the vein. For varicose veins in the legs, the use of compression or circulation socks can bring relief, as can keeping the feet elevated when possible.

For vaginal varicosities, compresses and sitz baths work well. Treat this sensitive area overnight by sleeping with a compress between your legs or inserting a tampon soaked in witch hazel. You can also apply tinctures of St. John's wort and yarrow to the area.

My top recommendation for treating varicose veins is to use a cool compress, which is astringent and soothing. Herbal teas that can be made into compresses for varicose veins include blackberry leaf, horse chestnut bark, peach leaf, plantain, St. John's wort, and witch hazel.

Herbal tea can support overall vein health. Rich in nutrients, rose hip tea is an excellent choice for anyone who has varicose veins.

Varicose Vein Salve

YIELD: 3 CUPS

1 cup	**shredded beeswax**
1 cup	**St. John's wort infused oil**
½ cup	**calendula-infused oil**
½ cup	**horse chestnut bark, leaves, and/or chopped green fruit, infused in oil**

Follow the method for making salves, page 80.

APPLICATION INSTRUCTIONS: Apply as needed to the area surrounding the vein or apply very lightly over the vein. Do not massage the vein or the area around it.

YEAST INFECTIONS

Yeast infections are typically caused by the fungus *Candida albicans* and affect the crotch area, skin folds, and armpits. Vaginal yeast infections are very common during pregnancy, perhaps more so than during any other time in life.

The way to rid yourself of a yeast infection is to avoid common triggers. A key step is limiting sugar in the diet; adding garlic, probiotics, and cultured foods can also be helpful. Other triggers for infection include antibiotic use, having a partner with an infection, and not showering. Having uncontrolled diabetes or an impaired immune system also escalates risk for infection.

Vaginal yeast infections are more likely to occur when there are changes in the type and amount of bacteria normally present in the vagina. This can be caused by douching, not having enough vaginal lubrication during sex, or having a lot of sex in a short period of time without showering.

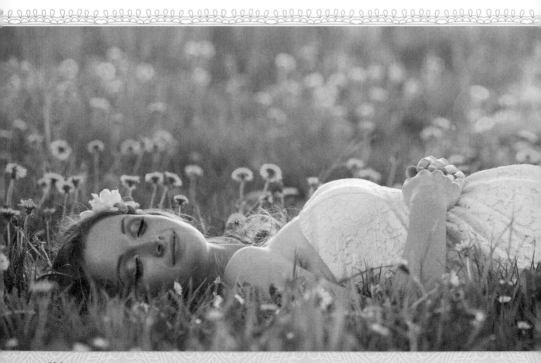

Yeast Wash Compress

YIELD: 1 COMPRESS

1 cup	**water**
1 teaspoon	**pau d'arco bark or powdered bark**
1 teaspoon	**raspberry leaves**
20 drops	**tea tree essential oil**

Follow the method for making a cool compress, page 85.

APPLICATION INSTRUCTIONS: Apply to the affected area.

Yeasty Powder

YIELD: ABOUT 4 TABLESPOONS

4 tablespoons	**acidophilus powder**
1 teaspoon	**pau d'arco powdered bark**

Put the acidophilus powder and pau d'arco in a small jar.

APPLICATION INSTRUCTIONS: Shake well before using. Dust the affected area.

VARIATION: Add 5 drops of tea tree essential oil.

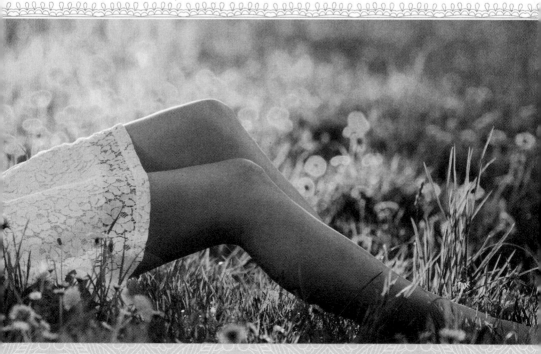

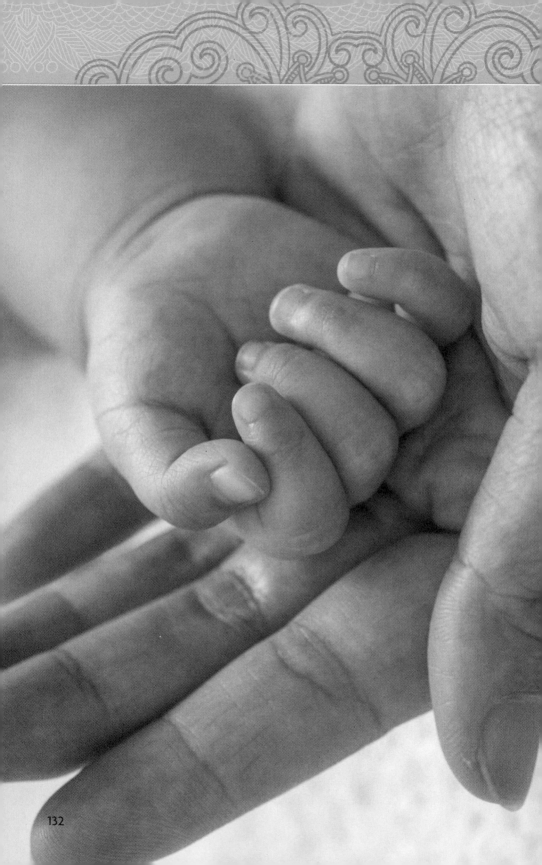

CHAPTER 7

Remedies for Labor and Delivery

During labor, herbal remedies can be a great alternative to pharmaceutical drugs, with appropriate usage and education. If you plan to use herbal remedies during labor, it is essential that you discuss your choices with your care provider, so they know your plan and can work with you.

As an herbalist, I'm wary of herbal practices that mimic modern medicine. Herbs should be used because they can bring about a desired and positive result. I also do not believe in starting herbs to assist labor five weeks before the due date (see box, page 134). This is a popular course of treatment in some circles, and I believe it is wrong.

Childbirth is a beautiful and natural process. Babies are born without herbs and without drugs every day. Any type of intervention is an intervention. Sometimes no intervention is needed. However, herbal therapies can be used to improve both comfort and safety during labor and childbirth. This chapter explores the three stages of labor—early, active, and transitional—as well as back labor, birth of the baby, and birth of the placenta. In addition, the characteristics of each stage are clearly described. Different herbal remedies can be helpful during each stage.

Labor can be induced using either herbs or pharmaceutical drugs. For many years, I have believed that labor should be induced using herbs at home only when it is beneficial to mother and baby, and never before forty-one weeks. In addition, labor should be induced only with professional guidance and oversight. Inducing labor prematurely can have negative outcomes for both the mother and the baby.

EARLY LABOR

Early labor is the phase that lasts the longest, spanning many hours and sometimes days. During this phase of labor, the cervix dilates up to 4 centimeters. Women in early labor may experience the following symptoms:

BLOODY SHOW. During early labor, most women will notice a bit of blood on the toilet paper when wiping after urination. Bleeding also may occur after a physical examination or intercourse.

EASILY MANAGEABLE CONTRACTIONS. Mild contractions start during this phase, often late. They typically last about thirty seconds with intervals of up to twenty minutes in between. You should be able to talk with ease during these contractions. All is well if the contractions are regular. Contact your care provider if they are not.

FLU-LIKE SYMPTOMS. Although it's normal to feel flu-like symptoms, such as chills, during this phase, contact your care provider if you have a fever.

FREQUENT, LOOSE BOWEL MOVEMENTS. It's normal to go to the bathroom a lot while your body is preparing for delivery. Some women claim their stools smell stronger and more acrid at this time.

MUCUS DISCHARGE. Some slightly bloody mucus is normal at this time. Discharge could also indicate that the mucus plug is being released; the mucus plug essentially creates a barrier over the cervix to protect the baby, and it is released shortly before labor. It can be released and regenerate a day or two before active labor begins. If the mucus discharge is green or really foul smelling, contact your care provider.

SPONTANEOUS RUPTURE OF MEMBRANES. Also known as water breaking, the spontaneous rupture of membranes doesn't usually happen during early labor. However, there is a small chance the water will break long before active labor begins, sometimes by a day or two.

ACTIVE LABOR

Active labor follows early labor and features many of the same characteristics but is more intense. During this phase, the cervix dilates between 5 and 8 centimeters.

BLOODY SHOW. Some slight blood or a combination of blood and mucus is likely to appear on the toilet paper after you urinate or on your bed linens in the morning.

CONTRACTIONS. During this phase, contractions become more frequent and more intense, and they also last longer. You will find it harder to talk during these contractions and may not be able to talk at all because the contractions may require your full attention.

SPONTANEOUS RUPTURE OF MEMBRANES. Your water is more likely to break during active labor than early labor. If the water is tarry and black or smells really bad, or you are less than thirty-seven weeks, contact your care provider.

BACK LABOR

Back labor is a common term used to describe intense pain in the lower back during labor; it is caused by the position of the baby. Often, but not always, back labor occurs when the baby is facing the mother's abdomen and the baby's head is putting pressure on the mother's tailbone. This position is called occiput posterior, and babies who are born this way are sometimes called sunny-side up.

Back labor can be managed and even reduced with herbal remedies. Following are a few that can help:

ARNICA GEL. Although arnica essential oil is not safe to use during pregnancy, gels that are made from arnica flowers can be used. Arnica gel is sold in most natural food stores and pharmacies.

RICE PACKS. Easy to make at home, rice packs can be heated and applied to the lower back for pain relief. To make a rice pack, fill a sock two-thirds full with uncooked rice. Tie off or sew the top shut, leaving room for the rice to move around. Alternatively, make a small rectangular pillow with cotton fabric by sewing three sides, filling the pillow two-thirds full with uncooked rice, and sewing the fourth side closed. To incorporate aromatherapy, add dried lavender flowers or peppermint leaves or a few drops of chamomile, lavender, peppermint, or sweet orange essential oil.

Warm the rice pack in the microwave for 45 to 90 seconds. Since microwaves vary in power, the exact time will depend on your microwave and how much rice was used. Alternatively, wrap the rice pack in foil and warm in the oven at 300 degrees F for 20 to 30 minutes. Check the temperature of the rice pack before using it; you do not want to burn yourself. If it is too hot, let it cool down until you can comfortably put it on your skin. If the pack is not hot enough, put it back in the microwave and heat it an additional 10 seconds at a time. A good practice is to place a towel between your skin and the rice pack.

Back Labor Liniment

YIELD: VARIABLE

2½ cups	**vodka**
3 ounces	**dried arnica flowers**
3 ounces	**dried lavender flowers**
3 ounces	**dried St. John's wort flowers**

Follow the method for making liniments, page 84.

APPLICATION INSTRUCTIONS: Apply to the affected area.

CAUTION: Do not apply to open wounds or broken skin.

TRANSITION

Transition, the shortest period of labor, can be a trying and tiring time for the mother. It is the time during which early labor transitions to active labor; during this span, cervical dilation increases to 10 centimeters. Transition labor is characterized by the following:

FEELINGS OF FEAR AND HELPLESSNESS. Your emotions at this time may be overwhelming. You may cry or even think you're not loved. It's good to be aware of this possibility and to alert the people who may be around you. They should be understanding if this occurs.

NAUSEA AND VOMITING. During this phase, it's common to vomit or feel like you have to. Be sure to have a receptacle, such as a basin or small wastebasket, close by. Sniffing ginger, peppermint, or spearmint essential oils can help fight nausea. Place a drop on a washcloth and hold it near your nose.

POSSIBLE URGE TO PUSH. You may feel like you're ready to push during transition, but wait.

PRESSURE ON VAGINA AND RECTUM. You will feel pressure in your vagina and rectum, and you may need to go to the bathroom.

SHAKING AND CHILLS. Although either of these may be alarming, feeling shaky or having the chills may occur during transition.

SPONTANEOUS RUPTURE OF MEMBRANES. This is the time when your water may break naturally. However, your care provider may have ruptured your membranes earlier if that is their practice.

STRONGER, MORE FREQUENT CONTRACTIONS. Contractions now will take all of your concentration and focus. In addition, because there is little time between contractions, you will have less opportunity to rest. Still, some women manage to sleep a minute at a time during transition.

Transition Room Spray

YIELD: 4 OUNCES

4 ounces	**water**
15 drops	**mandarin orange essential oil**
10 drops	**bergamot essential oil**
10 drops	**clary sage essential oil**
10 drops	**lavender essential oil**

Follow the method for making room sprays, page 78.

CAUTION: This is a powerful blend; when spraying, direct the mist away from you. Never spray yourself directly.

NOTE: This combination of essential oils is calming and grounding. It will help lift your spirits.

Transition Tincture Blend

YIELD: VARIABLE

1 part	**milky oats**
1 part	**motherwort leaves**
½ part	**lemon balm leaves**
1 part	**skullcap leaves**

Follow the method for making tinctures, page 83.

DOSAGE INSTRUCTIONS: Use 20 to 30 drops while in transition, if needed.

BIRTH OF THE BABY

After the transition, the birth begins. Between the phases, there may be a lull in contractions as your body prepares for the pushing phase. Some women use this time to nap. Many of the characteristics from the transition stage mark the birth phase as well, including increased pressure on the vagina and rectum and an increasing urge to push.

Crowning is the term used when the baby is starting to come out of the vagina. Because some women experience a burning sensation during crowning, this phase of birth is sometimes called "ring of fire." As soon as you feel this sensation, stop pushing! This is suggested so you do not tear tissues or increase the risk of needing an episiotomy. Relax and breathe deeply to lessen the sensation of burning. This feeling lasts only for a short time and is followed by a feeling of numbness, which occurs naturally and has an effect like an anesthetic. The baby's head is stretching the vaginal tissue so thin that the vaginal nerves are blocked.

Your doctor or midwife will tell you when to push and when not to push. Here are some ways to resist the urge to push:

- Lean back, go limp, and breathe deeply.
- Make a conscious effort to relax the muscles of the perineum. Breathe and imagine the area blooming, relaxing, and opening up.
- Allow your contractions to do the work at this time.
- Inhale lavender essential oil to promote relaxation.

When the baby is born, you don't need a specific herbal remedy. What the baby needs is to be held close to your body, to nurse, and to feel your touch. Babies want to be held and loved. Your care provider can do the newborn exam with the baby on you. If all is fine, continue to snuggle and breastfeed; ideally, you and the baby should have skin-to-skin contact. If an emergency occurs, most care providers will try to make the process efficient to get the baby back into your arms as quickly as possible.

After the birth, you may be hungry. Have a nourishing soup and tea for a lovely post-birth meal. But don't be surprised if you want a whole pizza!

BIRTH OF THE PLACENTA

After the birth of the baby comes the birth of the placenta. It can take between a few minutes and almost an hour for the placenta to detach. After the placenta is expelled, heavy bleeding, but not hemorrhaging, normally occurs.

If the placenta doesn't readily detach, it can become life threatening. After the placenta is delivered, the uterus contracts, which causes the blood vessels within it to constrict. When the placenta is retained, the uterus is incapable of performing this function. The blood vessels need to close off or they continue to bleed. This could cause a hemorrhage, and the mother could require a blood transfusion.

Within the birthing community, there are differing views about how to handle the birth of the placenta. Midwives do not use controlled cord traction to promote delivery of the placenta, although other caregivers might. This involves pulling on the umbilical cord and applying counterpressure to help deliver the placenta. I discourage this practice because pulling out the placenta before it has naturally detached from the uterus can cause hemorrhage. Some herbal tinctures that can help deliver the placenta naturally include angelica, blue cohosh, and raspberry leaf.

Here's what to expect when the placenta is delivered. You will feel a lull in contractions as your body waits to expel the placenta. You will then experience a slight urge to push as the placenta detaches fully, descends, and slips out of the vagina. You may not want to push out the placenta, as you will understandably feel exhausted already, but you must be ready to do as your caregiver advises. You will continue to need support through this phase of the birth. You may also experience some shaking and pain in the vagina, which will be especially tender at this time.

DELAYED PLACENTA

Different care providers will have different standards for how long it should take the placenta to come out naturally. When this time period has passed, caregivers may try different techniques to encourage the placenta to be born. For example, having the mother breastfeed during this time can stimulate placental delivery. In addition, the caregiver may suggest that the mother shift positions and become more upright.

There are a number of herbal remedies that can encourage delivery of the placenta. Following are some examples:

ANGELICA ROOT EXTRACT. Place a drop under your tongue and follow with a swallow of water.

FEVERFEW FLOWER INFUSION. This can be made when labor starts. Put 4 teaspoons of feverfew flowers in a quart jar, fill the jar with boiling water, and let sit at room temperature for 30 minutes. Put the lid on and refrigerate to keep fresh. Drink by the cupful.

HOT BASIL LEAF INFUSION. Follow the method for making infusions, page 81. Drink hot by the cupful.

A number of other herbal remedies are used only after the placenta has been delivered. Lady's Mantle Blend, Yarrow and Shepherd's Purse Tea, and Fleabane and Cinnamon Tincture Blend (remedies follow) are designed to stem bleeding, which is common after the placenta is delivered. Hemorrhage, however, is not common. If bleeding persists, seek emergency care.

Lady's Mantle Blend

YIELD: ½ CUP

3 tablespoons	**cotton root tincture**
2 tablespoons	**lady's mantle tincture**
1 tablespoon	**cinnamon tincture**
1 tablespoon	**honey**
1 tablespoon	**shepherd's purse tincture**

Combine all the ingredients in a clean 4-ounce bottle. Put the cap on the bottle and close tightly. Shake well to combine.

DOSAGE INSTRUCTIONS: Take 1 teaspoon of the blend orally as needed to stop bleeding. Use up to 8 teaspoons until the bleeding stops.

NOTE: Use only after the placenta has been delivered.

Yarrow and Shepherd's Purse Tea

YIELD: 4 CUPS PREPARED TEA

1 ounce	**dried yarrow flowers**
1 ounce	**dried shepherd's purse leaves**

Put the ingredients in a clean jar, put on the lid, and shake gently to combine. Put 8 tablespoons of the dried tea in a teapot. Pour 4 cups of boiling water over it. Cover and let steep for 30 minutes. Strain.

DOSAGE INSTRUCTIONS: Drink ¼ to 1 cup at a time, drinking up to 4 cups if needed to stop the bleeding.

NOTE: Use only after the placenta has been delivered. Sweeten lightly if desired.

Canada Fleabane and Cinnamon Tincture Blend

YIELD: ¼ CUP

3 tablespoons	**Canada fleabane tincture**
1 tablespoon	**cinnamon tincture**

Combine the ingredients in a clean 2-ounce bottle. Put the cap on the bottle and close tightly. Shake gently to combine.

DOSAGE INSTRUCTIONS: Take ½ teaspoon of the blend orally as needed.

MAXIMUM DOSAGE: Use up to 6 doses over 2 hours.

NOTE: Use only after the placenta has been delivered.

HEMORRHAGE

Hemorrhage after birth, or postpartum hemorrhage, is the loss of more than 500 milliliters (2.11 cups) of blood following vaginal delivery or 1,000 milliliters (about 5 cups) of blood following Cesarean section. Hemorrhage is the most common cause of perinatal maternal death in the industrialized world and is a major cause of maternal morbidity worldwide. It is a serious condition.

Most midwives and doctors have protocols they follow in the event of postpartum hemorrhage. Mothers who have hemorrhaged following prior births are at greater risk, so if you have had this in the past, make sure you tell your care provider. If you have a clotting disorder, please share that information also.

The primary causes of postpartum hemorrhage are uterine atony, trauma, retained placenta, and coagulopathy, commonly known as the "four Ts":

TONE. Uterine atony is the incapacity of the uterus to contract and clamp down on the blood vessels, which may lead to continuous bleeding. Retained placental tissue and infection may also cause uterine atony.

TRAUMA. Trauma from the delivery may tear tissue and vessels, potentially causing significant postpartum bleeding.

TISSUE. If any tissue from the placenta or fetus is not expelled, excessive bleeding may occur. This is why care providers make sure the placenta is intact after it is delivered.

THROMBIN. Hemorrhage can occur when the blood fails to clot. Thrombin is the enzyme that causes blood to clot or coagulate. Coagulopathies are diseases in which the blood fails to clot.

Hemorrhage is less likely to occur following a natural birth or a birth during which there is little intervention. To reduce the risk of hemorrhage, mothers are encouraged to eat a high-quality diet and get plenty of rest during pregnancy.

Following are some hemorrhage remedies that should be made ahead of time in case they are needed. Of course, a mother who is hemorrhaging should be monitored, and medical care should be administered. The mother should be transported to the hospital if the herbs are having no effect.

Infusion for Hemorrhage

YIELD: 2 CUPS DRIED TEA

1 cup	**dried nettles**
1 cup	**dried raspberry leaves**

Follow the method for making infusions, page 81.

DOSAGE INSTRUCTIONS: Drink 3 to 4 cups during the first 24 hours following delivery.

Extract Blend 1 for Hemorrhage

YIELD: ¼ CUP

2 tablespoons	**shepherd's purse seed, leaf, or flower extract**
2 tablespoons	**yarrow flower extract**

Put the ingredients in a small bottle. Put the cap on the bottle and close tightly. Shake gently to combine.

DOSAGE INSTRUCTIONS: Stir ½ teaspoon of the extract blend into warm water. Drink this amount every half hour.

Extract Blend 2 for Hemorrhage

YIELD: 3¼ TEASPOONS

1 teaspoon	**motherwort leaf extract**
1 teaspoon	**shepherd's purse seed, flower, or leaf extract**

| 1 teaspoon | **witch hazel leaf or bark extract** |
| ¼ teaspoon | **blue cohosh root extract** |

Put all the ingredients in a small bottle. Put the cap on the bottle and close tightly. Shake gently to combine.

DOSAGE INSTRUCTIONS: Take 2 droppersful orally. Follow with freshly made fruit or vegetable juice. Repeat in 1 minute, if needed, then again in 10 minutes.

Extract Blend 3 for Hemorrhage

YIELD: 2 TEASPOONS

| 1 teaspoon | **motherwort flower and leaf extract** |
| 1 teaspoon | **witch hazel leaf or bark extract** |

Put the ingredients in a small bottle. Put the cap on the bottle and close tightly. Shake gently to combine.

DOSAGE INSTRUCTIONS: Take 2 droppersful orally. Repeat in 10 minutes, if needed.

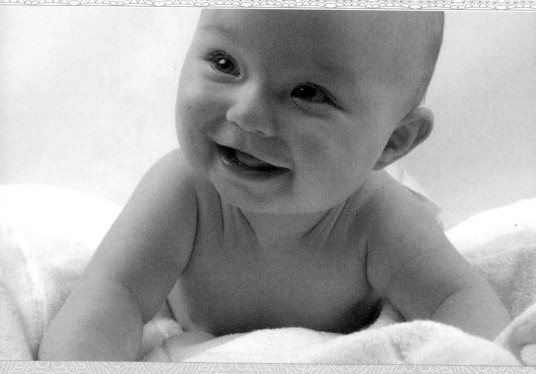

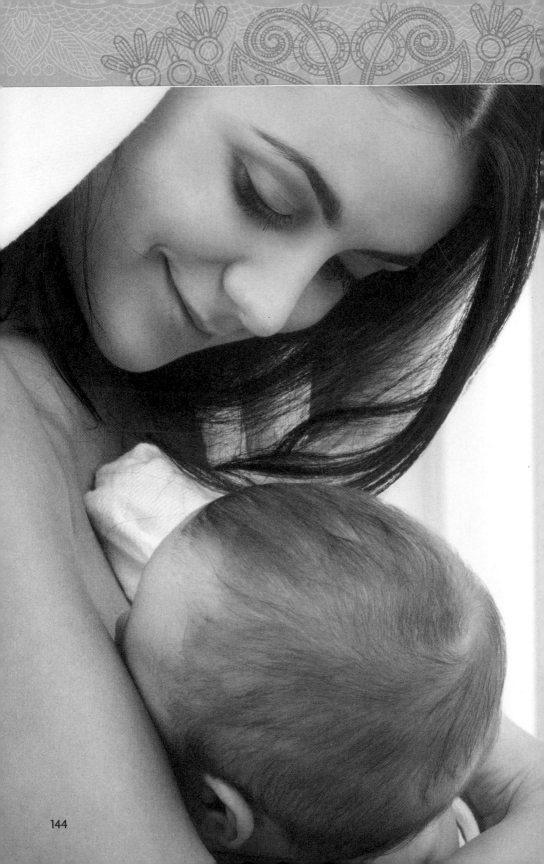

Remedies for Breast-feeding and Other Postpartum Concerns

Postpartum is the period from birth to six months, a time when the mother needs to take good care of herself and her baby. It's especially important during this time for the mother to get appropriate nutrition. Fresh fruits and vegetables are paramount, as are protein and whole grains. After all, a breastfeeding baby relies on the mother for nutrition. Nursing is one of the most powerful energy exchanges between two people. It creates an intense bond between mother and child that will last forever.

Breastfeeding is the best thing you can do for your baby. Nurse as frequently as possible, especially during the first few days after birth. During this time, your milk will contain colostrum, which is loaded with protein and antibodies that will help your baby's immune system. To fortify and increase your milk supply, drink plenty of pure water, herbal teas, and freshly made, vitamin-rich fruit and vegetable juices.

Herbal remedies can be helpful by providing nutrition and supporting successful breastfeeding, and these are two of the most important concerns during the postpartum period. Another priority is breast care, because soreness, cracked nipples, and even blockage and infection may occur.

In addition, postpartum depression is a serious and common issue. Here too, herbal remedies can be helpful, and a section in this chapter is devoted to this topic. During this time, try to surround yourself with people who can provide emotional and material support. Just be sure that anyone who comes to visit you and your baby washes up before touching either of you. To avoid contagions, try to keep the baby at home for at least ten days before venturing out.

A variety of other experiences, such as back pain and afterpain, are also common during the postpartum period. Other developments, such as prolapsed tissue in the vagina (cystocele) and rectum (rectocele) are less common but important to be aware of.

As is the case during all phases of pregnancy, you'll want to be mindful of what you see in your own body. Following are some of these:

BLEEDING. It is normal to have vaginal bleeding after delivery. This bloody vaginal discharge is commonly called lochia, and it typically persists for about six weeks, although some women have it for a much shorter time. Initially postpartum bleeding features bright red blood. It will later become more brown and then quite brown toward the end. During the first week, it will look like a normal menstrual period, for example, and the volume will lessen gradually. You will also notice some blood clots mixed in; this is normal. After the first week, the blood loss decreases until you experience bleeding similar to that of a very light period. As time goes on, this will change to spotting until the bleeding stops completely.

Use pads, not tampons, sponges, or diva cups, because of the increased risk of infection during the postpartum period. You will also want to refrain from sexual penetration or inserting anything in the vagina during this time.

BLOOD CLOTS. You may notice clots in your vaginal bleeding and experience cramping while breastfeeding. This is quite normal after delivery; however, call your care provider if you develop heavy bleeding, large clots (bigger than a ping pong ball), and have a fever of 100.4 F or higher.

POSTPARTUM HEMORRHAGE. If your postpartum bleeding increases or you soak a pad every hour or two, call your doctor to rule out postpartum hemorrhage. Postpartum hemorrhage can happen out of the blue. If your blood suddenly becomes bright red and your flow increases, it is an immediate sign that you need to slow down and take it easy. Contact your caregiver if the blood or any discharge has a foul odor or if you feel unwell, have loose stools, and are feverish.

SORENESS. Your perineum is likely to be sore for a couple of days to a couple of weeks; it will be sore longer if you have had an episiotomy. You may notice discomfort, especially when sitting or walking or during urination. To alleviate discomfort, fill a peri bottle (a perineal irrigation bottle, available online) with warm water and use as a rinse after urinating. While sitting on the toilet, use the bottle to squirt the water over the surface of the perineum, moving from front to back, before gently dabbing yourself dry. Also, try sitz baths and compresses.

THE FIRST FORTY-EIGHT HOURS

After the exertion of giving birth, a new mom needs to be replenished and refreshed. Herbal tea is just the ticket. I usually make You Rock! Mama Tea (remedy follows) by the gallon for clients to drink during the first forty-eight hours after birth. Mothers say they love the taste, and how it makes them feel. Relaxing and nutritious, it's packed with vitamin C and other vitamins, flavonoids, and minerals.

You Rock! Mama Tea

YIELD: ABOUT 4 CUPS DRIED TEA

1½ cups	**dried lemon balm leaves**
1 cup	**dried chamomile flowers**
1 cup	**dried hibiscus flowers**
½ cup	**dried rose petals**
2 tablespoons	**dried rose hips**
1 tablespoon	**dried lavender flowers**

Follow the method for making herbal tea, page 81. Put 5 to 10 tablespoons of dried tea in a large sun tea jar. Add 1 gallon of boiling water and let steep, covered, for 30 minutes. Strain before drinking.

DOSAGE INSTRUCTIONS: During the first 48 hours after delivery, drink 5 to 6 cups per day, or as needed.

NOTE: This herbal tea can be served warm or cold.

The postpartum period is a wonderful time to relax with some herbal tea, such as the You Rock! Mama Tea (page 147), which is designed to be used during the first forty-eight hours after birth. Drinking a variety of herbal teas throughout the postpartum period supplies you with minerals, vitamins, and other nutrients. In addition, herbal teas provide precious liquids, which promote the production of breast milk so you can successfully feed the baby. Although the time after birth can be extremely demanding, taking a few minutes to sit down and drink a cup of delicious tea gives you a bit of peace and a chance to catch your breath. Besides, discovering and making herbal tea blends is a fun and creative thing to do.

BREASTFEEDING AND MILK PRODUCTION

Breastfeeding mothers may feel anxiety about their ability to produce enough milk, but many have no problems. The keys to successful nursing are eating well, drinking enough fluids, relaxing, and persistence. This means putting the baby to your breast often, including throughout the night. Babies are not supposed to sleep through the night, so they need to be fed often and on demand. A baby who is gaining weight adequately is certainly getting enough milk, and a baby who is wetting six to eight diapers a day and pooping some is also being fed enough.

Anxiety and tension can inhibit a mother's ability to nurse; if this is true in your case, aromatherapy and herbal remedies can help you relax. Essential oils such as chamomile, clary sage, lavender, and sweet orange can be used in diffusers around the house to make you feel more relaxed and at peace. Alternatively, add a few drops to your bath, shampoo, lotion, or laundry soap. Herbs such as catnip, chamomile, hops, lemon balm, and lavender are gentle soothers to body and spirit, enabling you to slow down and be tranquil as you feed your baby. Drink lightly sweetened teas made from these herbs.

Basic, healthy behaviors encourage milk production. These include the following:

- Drink at least a half gallon of fluids daily. Herbal teas are an excellent choice. Limit caffeinated or sugary beverages, which can cause dehydration.

HERBS THAT ARE GALACTOGOGUES

Following is a list of some of the herbs that can help increase a breastfeeding mom's milk supply. These herbs can be taken as infusions (see method, page 81) or tinctures (dosages of 10 to 30 drops, 2 to 4 times per day):

- alfalfa
- blessed thistle leaves
- coriander
- dandelion root and leaves (see note, below)
- fennel
- fenugreek
- hops
- marshmallow root
- nettles
- oat straw
- oats
- raspberry leaves
- shatavari (see note, below)
- slippery elm bark
- spearmint

Note: Fresh dandelion leaves incorporated into salads, soups, and other dishes can be effective in promoting milk production. Shatavari, an herb that comes from Ayurvedic medicine, is a popular galactagogue in India and China.

- Eat enough calories (even more than during pregnancy!) to produce substantial amounts of milk. Increase your caloric intake about 500 calories.
- Feed your baby when your baby is asking to be fed. Some signs that the baby wants to eat include rooting at the breast, sucking on a fist, making noise, and eventually crying.
- Use breast massage to stimulate milk flow (see page 152).

Galactagogues are herbs and other substances that encourage the establishment of milk production as well as increase total volume. Most mothers do not need galactagogues, although some may have a genuinely low milk supply. Some working mothers use galactagogues to increase their output when pumping so they have milk for when they are not home. They may do this even though their supply is fine when the baby nurses.

In addition to herbs, beer has been discussed as an effective galactagogue over the years, but the evidence isn't conclusive. Besides, consuming alcohol when breastfeeding is discouraged. One alternative for nursing mothers is malta, a nonalcoholic beverage made from barley and hops that may be helpful in milk production.

Mother's Milk Tea

1 cup	**dried catnip**
1 cup	**dried chamomile flowers**
½ cup	**dried borage flowers and leaves**
¼ cup	**fennel seeds**
2 tablespoons	**dried lavender flowers**

Follow the method for making herbal teas as infusions, page 81. Use 1 tablespoon of dried tea per 1 cup of boiling water. Let steep for 10 minutes.

DOSAGE INSTRUCTIONS: Drink 1 cup, 2 to 3 times per day.

VARIATION: For a stronger tea, put ¼ cup of dried tea in a quart jar. Add boiling water and let steep, covered, for 20 minutes.

Mama Milk

1 cup	**dried nettles**
1 cup	**raspberry leaves**
½ cup	**blessed thistle leaves**
½ cup	**fennel seeds, crushed**
¼ cup	**fenugreek seeds, crushed**

Follow the method for making herbal tea, page 81. Pour 1 cup of water into a small saucepan and heat over medium heat until the water begins to simmer gently; if necessary, decrease the heat to medium-low to maintain a gentle simmer. Add 2 teaspoons of the dried tea, cover the saucepan, and simmer for 10 minutes. Strain before drinking.

DOSAGE INSTRUCTIONS: Drink 1 cup, 2 to 3 times per day.

NOTE: Although it's not necessary for most herbal teas, I like to let this one simmer on the stovetop to get the most benefit from the many leaves used.

Milk Seed Tea

YIELD: 2¼ CUPS DRIED TEA

1 cup	**red raspberry leaves**
½ cup	**aniseeds, crushed**
½ cup	**fennel seeds, crushed**
¼ cup	**caraway seeds, crushed**

Follow the method for making herbal teas as infusions, page 81.

DOSAGE INSTRUCTIONS: Drink 1 cup, 2 to 3 times per day.

Infusion to Relax a Breastfeeding Mom

YIELD: 4 TABLESPOONS FRESH, OR 8 TEASPOONS DRIED

1 tablespoon	**fresh borage, or 2 teaspoons dried**
1 tablespoon	**fresh clover leaves and flowers, or 2 teaspoons dried**
1 tablespoon	**fresh raspberry leaves, or 2 teaspoons dried**
1 tablespoon	**fresh rose hips, or 2 teaspoons dried**

Follow the method for making herbal tea, page 81. Use 1 tablespoon of fresh herbs or 2 teaspoons of dried herbs per 1 cup of water.

DOSAGE INSTRUCTIONS: Drink 1 cup, 2 to 3 times per day.

NOTE: This tea promotes relaxation but is also an excellent remedy for a mother who has a cold.

Tea for an Anxious Mother

YIELD: 3½ CUPS DRIED TEA

1 cup	**dried borage flowers and leaves**
1 cup	**dried motherwort leaves**
1 cup	**dried nettles**
½ cup	**dried peppermint leaves**

Follow the method for making herbal teas as infusions, page 81.

DOSAGE INSTRUCTIONS: Drink 1 cup, 2 to 3 times per day.

Massage Oil for Increasing Milk Production

YIELD: ABOUT 2 TABLESPOONS

2 tablespoons	**carrier oil** (see box, page 14)
15 drops	**clary sage, fennel, or geranium essential oil**

Follow the method for making blended and massage oils, page 79.

APPLICATION INSTRUCTIONS: Shake well before using. To massage your breasts, wash your hands with soap before starting but rinse well to avoid getting soap on your nipples. When massaging, use the flat part of the fingers and press firmly but gently. Start at the top of the breast and move in circles toward the center. After several seconds, move the fingers to a spot about one inch away and massage again. Repeat.

BREAST CARE DURING BREASTFEEDING

Breasts can take a beating during the postpartum phase. The most common complaints a breastfeeding mother might have include sore breasts and cracked nipples. More serious is a blocked duct or mastitis. From massage to herbal remedies, there are gentle and effective ways to keep your breasts healthy and productive.

Massage Oil for Sore Breasts

YIELD: ABOUT 3 TABLESPOONS

3 tablespoons	**carrier oil** (see box, page 14)
10 drops	**lavender essential oil**
10 drops	**Roman chamomile essential oil**
5 drops	**geranium essential oil**

Follow the method for making blended and massage oils, page 79.

APPLICATION INSTRUCTIONS: See instructions for Massage Oil for Increasing Milk Production, above.

Cracked Nipples

Cracked nipples are painful. For breastfeeding mothers who experience this condition, there are many solutions. One is to make sure the baby is latched on correctly and not taking too much of the breast into the mouth. Incorrect use of a breast pump may also result in cracked nipples. If you experience this side effect of breastfeeding or pumping, avoid creams, soaps, and even washing detergents that might cause irritation. In addition, always allow wet nipples to air-dry. And try some of the following natural treatments to relieve soreness and promote healing:

BREAST MILK. One of the simplest remedies for cracked nipples is to gently massage some of your own breast milk into the nipples and allow them to thoroughly air-dry.

COMPRESSES. Make compresses (see page 85) using either lemon balm or plantain and apply to the nipples.

EXPOSURE TO SUNLIGHT. Topless sunbathing for short periods of time (so you avoid sunburn to this delicate area) can help heal cracked nipples.

LANOLIN. Choose purified lanolin and apply gently to the nipples and surrounding skin.

PLANTAIN OINTMENT. Use a ready-made ointment or make one with plantain-infused oil (see page 81). Apply gently to the nipples and surrounding skin.

Cracked Nipple Massage Oil

YIELD: ABOUT 3 TABLESPOONS

3 tablespoons	**almond oil or olive oil**
1 teaspoon	**wheat germ oil or vitamin E oil**
10 drops	**calendula-infused oil**

Follow the method for making blended and massage oils, page 79.

APPLICATION INSTRUCTIONS: Shake well before using. Massage gently into the nipples using two fingers. Use a circular motion.

Blocked Duct

A blocked duct is a painful, swollen, firm mass in the breast. The skin covering the blocked duct is often quite red, which also occurs during mastitis (see page 154). In fact, if it's not resolved, a blocked duct can lead to mastitis, which is even more painful. Warmth, provided by a bath or shower, heating pad, or compress can help provide relief. Following are some additional tips to clear a blocked duct:

BREASTFEEDING. Nursing your baby frequently is the best way to clear a blocked duct.

EMPTYING THE BREAST. A blocked duct is more likely to occur in a breast that has not been completely emptied. Gently but firmly compress the breast to make sure it is emptied, but don't do so when the baby is drinking.

HOT COMPRESSES. Compresses made of calendula, comfrey, parsley, and plantain are often helpful. These compresses should be hot, but make sure they are not too hot; you don't want to scald yourself. Wait one half-hour after using a compress to nurse. In addition, gently but thoroughly rinse the beasts before nursing.

MARSHMALLOW COMPRESS OR SOAK. Soak the affected breast in a decoction of marshmallow root. Alternatively, apply a compress made from marshmallow root.

Mastitis

Mastitis is inflammation of the mammary glands inside the breast, and it can become serious rather quickly. Mastitis usually affects women who are breastfeeding. Hence, it is often referred to as lactation mastitis.

Mastitis can occur as a result of an infection or a blocked milk duct. When milk is left pooled in the sacs, particularly if the breast has been partly emptied, it becomes a breeding ground for bacteria, which can lead to infection. Mastitis is more likely during illness and increased stress.

The following indicators of mastitis can develop quickly. Contact your caregiver immediately if you experience these primary symptoms:

- an area of the breast becomes red
- the affected area of the breast hurts, especially when touched
- the sore area of the breast is hot to the touch
- there is a burning sensation

Sometimes the indicators listed above are accompanied by the following additional symptoms:

- anxiety, feeling stressed
- body aches and pains
- chills
- elevated body temperature
- fatigue
- malaise
- shivering

If you experience mastitis, seek help from your caregiver. In addition, be sure to get plenty of rest and eat a nutritious diet. The following strategies can also help:

CALENDULA COMPRESS. Use calendula or other antimicrobial and vulnerary herbs to make a warm compress.

CLEAN NIPPLES. Keep the nipples and surrounding skin clean.

A number of herbs are not considered safe either to use topically or take internally while nursing. Because certain herbs can harm the nursing mother, the baby, or both, be sure to research any herb before using it. Following is a partial list of some of the common herbs that should not be used when you're breastfeeding:

- bladderwrack
- buckthorn
- butterbur
- chaparral
- coltsfoot
- dong quai
- elecampane
- ephedra; ma huang *(see note)*
- ginseng
- kava kava
- rhubarb
- senna
- star anise
- uva ursi
- wormwood

Following is a list of herbs that should not be taken internally when breastfeeding:

- black walnut
- herb Robert
- periwinkle
- yarrow

Note: Ephedra and ma huang are used for many purposes but are best known in recent years as weight-loss aids. Avoid all diet and weight-loss supplements, herbal or otherwise, during the postpartum period and beyond.

A number of culinary herbs, such as oregano and thyme, are fine to use as food seasonings during the postpartum period, provided they're not consumed in large quantities. For a list of herbs that are safe for culinary use, see page 75.

HYDRATION. Drink plenty of fluids, such as herbal teas and water, to stay adequately hydrated and flush toxins from your system.

PAIN-RELIEVING OIL. Mastitis may cause the shoulder and chest muscles to become sore. If that happens, use a few drops of grapefruit, lavender, or peppermint essential oil added to St. John's wort infused oil. Apply topically by rubbing gently into the sore muscles.

UNHURRIED NURSING. Take your time when nursing and try to stay relaxed.

POSTPARTUM DEPRESSION

Postpartum depression is associated with the rapid change of hormones in the mother's body after she gives birth, and it can also occur following miscarriage and stillbirth. Many women experience postpartum depression, but the good news is that the condition can be treated and managed. Make sure you talk to your care provider if you suspect depression is a problem for you. If you have thoughts about harming yourself or your baby, find help immediately.

Because hormonal fluctuations after birth cause postpartum depression, behaviors and herbal remedies that rebalance hormones can help prevent or resolve it. My first suggestion for preventing postpartum depression is breastfeeding, which helps moderate hormonal swings and increases the body's endorphin and oxytocin levels. My other top suggestions are to get plenty of rest, eat right, and seek support from loved ones In addition, I suggest using the following herbs to rebalance your hormones:

- chamomile
- ginseng
- hops
- lemon balm leaves
- motherwort
- oats
- skullcap
- St. John's wort

Symptoms of postpartum depression include unhappiness, loss of interest in activities you once enjoyed, feelings of worthlessness and guilt, and excessive anxiety about the baby's health. Specific herbs can be used to treat these particular aspects of postpartum depression:

LOW MOOD, UNHAPPINESS. Use borage, rosemary, and St. John's wort extracts.

LOSS OF INTEREST IN USUALLY PLEASURABLE ACTIVITIES. Take relaxing baths and enjoy massages with oils that contain invigorating essential oils, such as grapefruit, peppermint, rosemary, and tangerine. To make a massage oil, add a few drops of essential oil to 1 tablespoon of carrier oil (see box, page 14).

FEELINGS OF WORTHLESSNESS OR GUILT. Drink herbal teas made with hibiscus, lemon balm, rooibos, and rose hips, alone or in combination.

EXCESSIVE ANXIETY OVER BABY'S HEALTH. Use lemon balm or motherwort tincture to help relieve anxiety.

Tea Blend for Depression and Fatigue

YIELD: 2½ CUPS DRIED TEA

1 cup	**dried chamomile flowers**
1 cup	**valerian root**
½ cup	**hops**

Follow the method for making teas as infusions, page 81. Let steep for 10 to 15 minutes.

DOSAGE INSTRUCTIONS: Drink 1 cup, 2 to 3 times per day.

Postpartum Tea

2 cups	**water**
½ teaspoon	**licorice root**
1 teaspoon	**dried raspberry leaves**
1 teaspoon	**dried rosemary leaves**
1 teaspoon	**dried skullcap leaves**
1 teaspoon	**dried spearmint leaves**

Put the water and licorice in a small saucepan over medium heat until the water begins to simmer gently; if necessary, decrease the heat to medium-low to maintain a gentle simmer. Let simmer, partially covered, for 20 minutes. Remove from the heat and add the raspberry, rosemary, skullcap, and spearmint. Let steep, covered, for 10 minutes.

DOSAGE INSTRUCTIONS: Drink 1 to 2 cups per day. More than that is not recommended.

Postpartum Room Spray

4 ounces	**water**
10 drops	**clary sage essential oil**
10 drops	**grapefruit essential oil**
10 drops	**tangerine essential oil**

Follow the method for making room sprays, page 78.

VARIATIONS: Instead of the essential oils listed above, use 10 drops of narcissus essential oil and 10 drops of neroli essential oil. Another variation is to use 10 drops of geranium essential oil and 5 drops of mandarin essential oil.

Postpartum Massage Oil 1

¼ cup	**carrier oil** (see box, page 14)
10 drops	**grapefruit essential oil**
10 drops	**neroli essential oil**
5 drops	**geranium essential oil**

Follow the method for making blended and massage oils, page 79.

APPLICATION INSTRUCTIONS: Shake well before using. Use as needed.

Postpartum Massage Oil 2

YIELD: ¼ CUP

¼ cup	**carrier oil** (see box, page 14)
10 drops	**bergamot essential oil**
5 drops	**clary sage essential oil**
2 drops	**rose essential oil**

Follow the method for making blended and massage oils, page 79.

APPLICATION INSTRUCTIONS: Shake well before using. Use as needed.

OTHER POSTPARTUM REMEDIES

Many of the discomforts that occur during pregnancy have a similar variation during the postpartum period. These include anemia; backache; contractions, or afterpains as they're called following birth; and incontinence. Other conditions are unique to this period and include prolapse and tissue injuries that follow birth and episiotomy. Remedies for all these conditions follow, but remember that they're designed specifically for use *after* the baby is born. Do not use postpartum remedies during pregnancy or labor because they may contain essential oils or herbs that are not safe to use during these times.

Afterpains

Afterpains, which occur as the uterus contracts and returns to its normal size, often are not discussed with first-time mothers, and these contractions can come as a surprise. During pregnancy, the uterus expands to twenty-five times its original size; the post-birth contractions shrink the uterus back down to size. Most of these contractions occur during the first hours after birth, but noticeable contractions can persist for a few days. After that the uterus may continue to contract for up to six weeks, although these contractions are likely to be quite mild and go relatively unnoticed. Breastfeeding will cause the uterus to contract back to its normal size more quickly, hastening recovery.

Severe cramping accompanied by uterine tenderness is not normal. If you notice these or any of the following symptoms, which can indicate a serious uterine infection, seek medical care immediately:

- a uterine area that feels "hot"
- a full feeling in the uterine area

- fever
- foul-smelling discharge

Aromatherapy, compresses, herbal extracts, massage oils, and hot teas are all good remedies for afterpains. Following are some suggestions:

AROMATHERAPY. Inhale jasmine absolute, which serves the dual purpose of encouraging uterine contractions and providing relief for afterpains.

HERBAL EXTRACTS. Try the following herbal extracts or combine them in an extract blend: black haw, cotton bark, and cramp bark. Take 20 drops orally, 2 to 3 times per day.

MASSAGE OIL OR LOTION. Make a massage oil by combining 1 table-spoon of carrier oil (see box, page 14) with a few drops of jasmine absolute. Alternatively, add a few drops of jasmine absolute to a small amount of your favorite lotion. Apply to the abdomen.

RICE PACK. Make a rice pack (see page 135) and apply it to the abdomen. Some helpful medicinal herbs to include in the rice pack are dried lavender, peppermint, and rosemary.

WARM COMPRESS. To make a simple compress, fill a large bowl with warm water. Add 10 drops of frankincense essential oil and 10 drops of lavender essential oil. Soak a washcloth in the mixture, wring it out, and apply it to the abdomen. Repeat as the washcloth cools.

Catnip Tea

YIELD: 1 CUP PREPARED TEA

| 1 cup | **boiling water** |
| 1 tablespoon | **dried catnip** |

Follow the method for making herbal teas as infusions, page 81. Cover and let steep for 10 to 15 minutes. Strain before drinking.

DOSAGE INSTRUCTIONS: Drink 1 cup of warm tea, 2 to 3 times per day.

NOTE: Sweeten lightly if desired.

VARIATION: Use 1½ teaspoons of dried catnip and 1½ teaspoons of dried chamomile flowers instead of 1 tablespoon of catnip.

MOTHERWORT TEA: Stir in 1 teaspoon of motherwort tincture after the Catnip Tea has been steeped and strained.

Chamomile Tea

YIELD: 1 CUP PREPARED TEA

1 cup **boiling water**

1 tablespoon **dried chamomile flowers**

Follow the method for making herbal teas as infusions, page 81. Cover and let steep for 10 to 15 minutes. Strain before drinking.

DOSAGE INSTRUCTIONS: Drink 1 cup of warm tea, 1 to 4 times per day.

NOTE: Sweeten lightly if desired.

Massage Oil for Afterpains

YIELD: 3 OUNCES

3 ounces **light carrier oil** (see box, page 14)

10 drops **jasmine absolute**

10 drops **lavender essential oil**

Follow the method for making blended and massage oils, page 79.

APPLICATION INSTRUCTIONS: Shake well before using. Apply to the abdomen as needed.

Tincture Blend for Afterpains

YIELD: VARIABLE

2 parts **motherwort leaves**

1 part **chamomile flowers**

1 part **cramp bark**

1 part **lavender flowers**

1 part **lemon balm leaves**

Follow the method for making tinctures, page 83.

DOSAGE INSTRUCTIONS: Take 20 to 30 drops orally, 2 to 3 times per day.

Anemia

Anemia is a condition in which iron levels in the blood are low; it can occur both during and after pregnancy. For a full explanation of anemia, see page 91. The following are remedies for anemia during the postpartum period.

Anemia Tea for the Postpartum Period

YIELD: 2½ CUPS DRIED TEA

1 cup	**dried peppermint leaves**
½ cup	**dried dandelion leaves**
½ cup	**dried nettles**
½ cup	**yellow dock root**

Follow the method for making herbal tea, page 81. Pour 1 cup of water into a small saucepan and heat over medium heat until the water begins to simmer; if necessary, decrease the heat to medium-low to maintain a gentle simmer. Add 2 teaspoons of the dried tea, cover the saucepan, and simmer for 20 minutes. Remove from the heat and let steep, covered, for another 20 minutes. Strain before drinking.

DOSAGE INSTRUCTIONS: Drink 1 cup, 3 to 5 times per day.

NOTE: Do not use during pregnancy. For anemia remedies that can be used during pregnancy, see page 91.

Anemia Tincture Blend for the Postpartum Period

YIELD: VARIABLE

1 part	**dried alfalfa leaves**
1 part	**dried nettles**
1 part	**yellow dock root**
½ part	**kelp** (see note)

Follow the method for making tinctures, page 83.

DOSAGE INSTRUCTIONS: Take 20 drops orally, 2 to 3 times per day.

NOTE: Kelp is a sea vegetable; dried kelp is sold online or at natural food stores. Do not use this tincture blend during pregnancy. For anemia remedies that can be used during pregnancy, see page 91.

Back Pain

Postpartum back pain is fairly common. Many women feel exhausted and sore during the first weeks after birth. Also hormones loosen ligaments both in the abdomen and back during labor. So in addition to having weaker back muscles, you have less support for the back because the abdominal muscles have also been stretched and weakened. The result is back pain.

Some practices during and after pregnancy can help you avoid back pain. Keep the following in mind:

CORRECT POSTURE. Be mindful of your posture throughout your pregnancy. You may be less likely to maintain a straight back as your abdomen grows and your gait changes, and this can contribute to back pain. In addition, try not to sit hunched over when breastfeeding.

PROPER LIFTING. Remember to bend from the knees, not the back, when you lift your baby.

Back Liniment

YIELD: ½ CUP

½ cup	**St. John's wort tincture**
10 drops	**rosemary essential oil**
5 drops	**eucalyptus essential oil**

Follow the method for making liniments, page 80.

APPLICATION INSTRUCTIONS: Shake well before using. Apply to the affected area.

VARIATION: Put ¼ cup of the liniment in a medium bowl. Wet a washcloth with hot water and soak the washcloth in the liniment mixture. Wring out the washcloth and apply it like a compress to the affected area.

Backache Massage Oil

YIELD: 4 OUNCES

2 ounces	**plantain-infused oil**
2 ounces	**St. John's wort infused oil**
10 drops	**peppermint essential oil**
5 drops	**juniper essential oil or rosemary essential oil**
5 drops	**lavender essential oil**

Follow the method for making blended and massage oils, page 79.

APPLICATION INSTRUCTIONS: Shake well before using. Apply as needed.

Carpal Tunnel Syndrome

Carpal tunnel syndrome may occur during pregnancy. Although it usually resolves after pregnancy, some discomfort may linger during the postpartum period. See remedies for carpal tunnel syndrome on pages 98 to 100.

Prolapses: Cystocele and Rectocele

Two types of prolapses can occur during the postpartum period. A prolapse occurs when an organ or body part slips out of its usual position, invading another area. Two types of prolapses can affect the vaginal area: a cystocele involves the bladder and a rectocele involves the rectal wall. Although these prolapses are fairly common, many women are unaware of them. I have been surprised to learn how many of my students have experienced one type of prolapse or the other without advance notice that they might result from childbirth.

In addition to everything else a new mother needs to know, it's important to be aware of the potential for prolapses. If you suspect you have a prolapse, seek care.

Cystocele

A cystocele, also called a prolapsed bladder, occurs when the wall between the bladder and vagina weakens and stretches, allowing the bladder to bulge into the vaginal area. A cystocele may result from the excessive straining that can occur during childbirth. Older women and those who have given birth to several children are more likely to develop a cystocele. In part, this is because estrogen levels, which can help protect against prolapse, decrease with age. Chronic constipation and weight lifting can also result in cystocele.

Connective Tissue Tea

YIELD: ABOUT ¾ CUP

5 tablespoons	**dried horsetail**
5 tablespoons	**dried oat straw**
2 tablespoons	**marshmallow root**
1 tablespoon	**dried alfalfa leaves**
1 tablespoon	**dried dandelion leaves**

Follow the method for making herbal teas as infusions, page 81.

DOSAGE INSTRUCTIONS: Drink 2 to 3 cups per day.

Many women who have a cystocele use a vaginal pessary, which is a plastic or rubber ring that is inserted into the vagina to help support the bladder. Herbs that strengthen connective tissues, such as horsetail, can also be helpful when incorporated into tea blends, including Connective Tissue Tea (see page 163).

Rectocele

A rectocele is a posterior prolapse; it occurs when the rectal wall bulges into the vaginal cavity. Although rectoceles can follow childbirth, they occur for other reasons as well. Any woman can have one.

A minor prolapse may not even be noticeable; if you have a larger rectocele, you can actually feel the bulge. Minor rectoceles do not need any medical treatment and eventually resolve themselves. Make an appointment with your doctor, however, if you notice any of the following signs, which may indicate a major prolapse:

BULGING TISSUE. A bothersome bulge of tissue may protrude from your vaginal opening when you strain. To do a self-examination, lay on the bed with your knees up and apart or sit on the toilet with knees apart; in either position, bear down. If you have a large rectocele, you will be able to use your hand to feel it protruding from your vagina.

PERSISTENT CONSTIPATION. You may have a large rectocele if methods to relieve constipation are not working. That's because the rectocele physically impedes the bowel movement. In fact, some women find that the stool seems to settle into the bulging area; manually applying counterpressure to the bulge from inside the vagina can release the stool.

UNCOMFORTABLE SEX. A large rectocele can cause rubbing or friction during sex, especially if you have not evacuated your bowels beforehand.

Tears and Episiotomies

Following a vaginal delivery, vaginal tissues will be sore, swollen, and torn. Sitz baths and other topical treatments, including compresses and peri-bottle rinses, are essential for providing relief and promoting healing.

It's normal for vaginal tissue to tear during birth. Until recently, it was common practice to routinely perform an episiotomy, an incision made in the skin and muscles between the vagina and the anus, to enlarge the vaginal opening during childbirth. The procedure was done to avoid natural tearing and, it was thought, to prevent damage to the baby's head. Present research shows that the procedure is necessary only in rare cases of fetal distress.

If possible, decline an episiotomy in favor of letting the tissues tear naturally. Studies show that natural tears generally heal more quickly than surgical ones, which cut through deeper layers of tissue. To treat natural tears, practitioners will often use seaweed, suture glue, and suture tape instead of stitches. (Without stitches, the perineum will heal more readily and less painfully.) It's also a good idea to apply ice immediately after the repair to decrease swelling.

Several natural methods can be used to speed healing and decrease pain. Following are some suggestions:

BED REST. Limiting your activity will help tears to heal, especially more severe tears.

COMFREY TEA. Drink fresh tea made from comfrey leaves (see method, page 81).

FRESH AIR AND SUNLIGHT. Get plenty of fresh air and go outside into the sunshine if possible.

PERINEUM WASH. Make a perineum wash by adding ¼ cup of lavender infusion to 1 cup of warm water. Add a drop of tea tree or patchouli essential oil. Use a peri bottle to rinse after urinating or simply use the wash anytime to soothe swollen and sore tissues.

VITAMIN E. Take 600 milligrams per day.

WITCH HAZEL PADS. Cooling and excellent for reducing swelling, witch hazel pads are sold in pharmacies and convenient to have on hand. Put three or four of the small, round witch hazel pads on a sanitary napkin pressed securely into your panties to ensure the witch hazel makes full contact with the perineum.

Hydrotherapy using both warm and cold water stimulates blood flow, which in turn promotes healing. During the postpartum period, your best friends may be your sitz-bath pans and your peri bottle, both of which can be used to provide relief to a sore and bruised perineum. See page 87 for general directions for making a sitz bath; in addition, four sitz-bath remedies follow. Simply make the herbal infusions as directed and use them in a sitz bath. If you prefer, any of the infusions can be used to make compresses or can be poured into a peri bottle and used to rinse the perineum.

CAUTION: If you have stitches, take only one sitz bath per day. Otherwise, use the baths, compresses, and rinses as needed to provide relief.

Two excellent essential oils to use for sitz baths are cypress and lavender. On page 166 is a list of herbs that are good choices for sitz baths. Those marked with an asterisk work well for severe tears as well as more minor tears and damage:

- aloe vera gel (*taken directly from fresh leaves*)
- calendula flowers
- chaparral*
- chickweed
- comfrey leaves*
- gotu kola*
- horse chestnut*
- horsetail*
- lavender flowers
- marshmallow root*
- oak bark
- plantain leaves
- rosemary
- St. John's wort flowers*
- white oak bark*
- witch hazel leaves or bark
- yarrow flowers

Epi-Sitz Blend

YIELD: ENOUGH FOR 1 SITZ BATH

3 cups	**simmering water**
4 tablespoons	**calendula flowers**
2 tablespoons	**comfrey leaves**
2 tablespoons	**St. John's wort**
4 drops	**lavender essential oil**
2 drops	**cypress essential oil**

Pour the water into a medium saucepan and bring to a simmer over medium heat. Remove from the heat and add the calendula, comfrey, and St. John's wort. Cover and let steep for 20 minutes. Strain and pour into a shallow bath. Add the lavender and cypress essential oils and mix well to disperse.

USAGE INSTRUCTIONS: Soak the vaginal area for about 20 minutes.

Postpartum Sitz Bath 1

YIELD: ENOUGH FOR 6 SITZ BATHS

2 cups	**sea salt**
1 cup	**dried calendula flowers**
1 cup	**rolled oats**
1 cup	**dried witch hazel leaves**
1 cup	**dried yarrow flowers**

Follow the method for making infusions, page 81, using about 1 cup of the herbal blend per 6 quarts of boiling water. Strain and pour into a shallow bath.

USAGE INSTRUCTIONS: Soak the vaginal area for about 20 minutes.

VARIATION: Use the infusion to make warm compresses or in a peri-bottle rinse.

Postpartum Sitz Bath 2

1 cup	**dried calendula flowers**
1 cup	**dried plantain leaves**
1 cup	**sea salt**
½ cup	**dried lavender flowers**
½ cup	**dried rosemary leaves**
½ cup	**dried shepherd's purse leaves**

Follow the method for making infusions, page 81, using about 1 cup of the herbal blend per 6 quarts of boiling water. Strain and pour into a shallow bath.

USAGE INSTRUCTIONS: Soak the vaginal area for about 20 minutes.

VARIATION: Use the infusion to make warm compresses or in a peri-bottle rinse.

Postpartum Sitz Bath 3

YIELD: ENOUGH FOR 4 TO 5 SITZ BATHS

1 cup	**dried plantain flowers**
½ cup	**dried burdock root**
½ cup	**dried calendula flowers**
½ cup	**dried comfrey leaves**
½ cup	**dried yarrow flowers**
¼ cup	**dried lady's mantle flowers and leaves**
¼ cup	**dried lemon balm leaves**
¼ cup	**dried violet flowers and leaves**

Follow the method for making infusions, page 81, using about 1 cup of the herbal blend per 6 quarts of boiling water. Strain and pour into a shallow bath.

USAGE INSTRUCTIONS: Soak the vaginal area for about 20 minutes.

VARIATIONS:

- Add ½ cup of sea salt to the herb mix.
- Use the infusion to make warm compresses or in a peri-bottle rinse.

Urinary Incontinence

Urinary incontinence is the loss of control of the bladder, and it can mean involuntarily leaking urine after childbirth when the muscles of the pelvic floor are weakened. This leakage can last for weeks to months. If you experience it, especially for a long period of time, talk to your doctor or a urologist.

As a temporary measure, wear pads or liners during the postpartum period to collect the urine. For long-term benefits, do exercises that will strengthen the pelvic floor.

Don't be tempted to restrict fluid intake during this time; in fact, it's more important than ever that you stay hydrated, especially if you're breastfeeding. Drink plenty of water and freshly made juices that are not likely to irritate your urinary tract, such as apple, blueberry, and cranberry juice. In addition, because constipation can be a contributing factor to incontinence, include fiber-rich fruits, vegetables, and grains in your diet.

Several herbs can be helpful in treating urinary incontinence. These include the following:

- cleavers
- corn silk
- couch grass
- dandelion leaves
- devil's claw
- horsetail
- marshmallow root
- parsley (except if breastfeeding)
- St. John's wort

One side effect of urinary incontinence is irritated skin. Topical treatments, including salves and dusting powders, can provide relief. A salve containing calendula, comfrey, and St. John's wort is a good choice. Dusting powders are soothing and provide a protective barrier. After having an accident, gently wipe the skin around the groin area with cider vinegar before applying (or reapplying) a topical remedy.

Dusting Powder 1

YIELD: 3½ CUPS

1½ cups	**cornstarch**
1 cup	**bentonite clay**
1 cup	**finely powdered herb, such as dried chamomile, lavender, or sandalwood**
3 to 5 drops	**lavender essential oil**

Put the cornstarch and clay in a medium bowl and whisk until well combined. Stir in the powdered herb and essential oil. Cover and let sit for 1 hour before transferring to a shaker jar.

USAGE INSTRUCTIONS: Shake before using. Sprinkle as needed to lightly cover sensitive areas, such as the inner thigh, that frequently come into contact with urine.

Dusting Powder 2

YIELD: 1 CUP

½ cup	**cornstarch**
½ cup	**white clay**
1 tablespoon	**finely powdered herb, such as chamomile or lavender** (see note)

Put the cornstarch and clay in a medium bowl and whisk until well combined. Stir in the powdered herb and transfer to a shaker jar.

USAGE INSTRUCTIONS: Shake before using. Sprinkle as needed to lightly cover sensitive areas, such as the inner thigh, that frequently come into contact with urine.

NOTE: Use any powdered herb that has a scent that you like.

Tonic Tea for Urinary Incontinence

YIELD: 2 CUPS DRIED TEA

½ cup	**couch grass root**
½ cup	**dandelion root, or 1 cup dried dandelion leaves**
½ cup	**marshmallow root**
½ cup	**dried parsley leaves** (see caution)

Follow the method for making teas as decoctions, page 81.

DOSAGE INSTRUCTIONS: Drink 2 to 3 cups per day.

CAUTION: Omit parsley if you're breastfeeding.

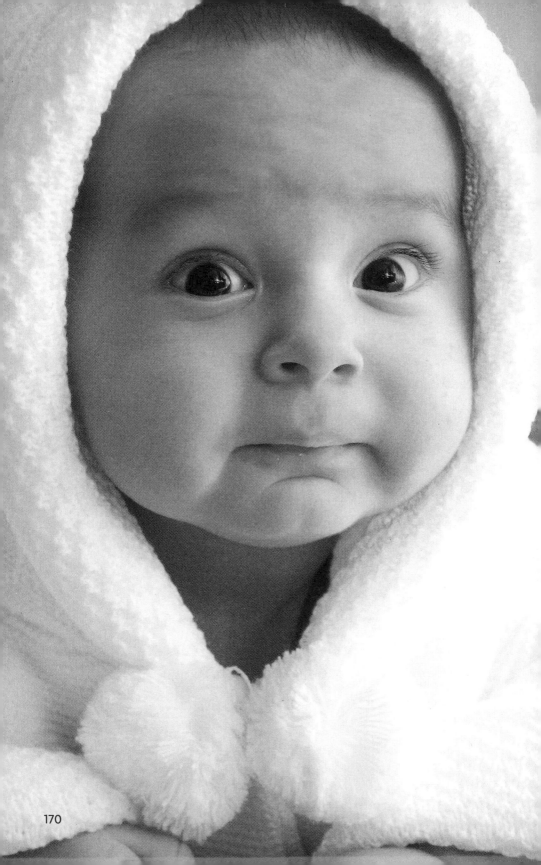

Glossary

Following are some medical terms used in this book:

Abortifacient. An abortifacient induces abortion or strong uterine contractions.

Acrid. Acrid describes a substance that has a bitter taste and could cause a sensation of heat and irritation when applied to the skin.

Alkaloids. Alkaloids are physiologically active compounds in plants that should be avoided because they affect bodily functions in the mother and fetus.

Alterative. An alterative modifies a condition by producing a steady change toward the renewal of health.

Analgesic. An analgesic relieves or diminishes pain.

Antianxiety. Any substance that has an antianxiety effect is one that prevents or relieves anxiety.

Antibacterial. An antibacterial combats bacterial infection.

Antibiotic. An antibiotic destroys, limits, or slows the growth of microorganisms.

Antifungal. An antifungal combats fungal infection.

Antihistamine. An antihistamine is used to counteract histamine, particularly when treating allergies.

Anti-inflammatory. An anti-inflammatory prevents or reduces inflammation.

Antimicrobial. An antimicrobial inhibits the growth of microorganisms.

Antinausea. Any substance that has an antinausea effect is one that prevents or relieves nausea.

Antiseptic. An antiseptic prevents the growth of microorganisms.

Antispasmodic. An antispasmodic prevents or allays spasms or cramps.

Antiviral. An antiviral is a substance that is effective against viruses.

Aphrodisiac. An aphrodisiac stimulates the sex organs.

Aromatic. An aromatic is an agent that emits a fragrant smell and produces a pungent taste. It is used chiefly to make other medicines more palatable.

Astringent. An astringent causes a contraction of tissues.

Demulcent. A demulcent is a soothing substance used to relieve internal inflammations. It provides a protective coating and allays irritation of the membranes.

Diuretic. A diuretic promotes secretions of the urinary system, aiding the elimination of excess fluid as well as toxins.

Emmenagogue. An emmenagogue acts upon the reproductive system, strengthening and balancing the cellular tissues by regulating the body's hormonal flow.

Emollient. An emollient soothes and softens the external skin surfaces and promotes healing.

Episiotomy. An episiotomy is a surgical cut made near the vagina during childbirth.

Expectorant. An expectorant promotes the excretion of sputum and is typically used to treat coughs.

Galactagogue. A galactagogue promotes the secretion of milk from the nursing breast.

Hypnotic. A hypnotic is capable of inducing sleep or hypnotic feelings.

Laxative. A laxative is used to promote a bowel movement.

Mucilage. A mucilage is a gelatinous substance that soothes inflammation.

Narcotics. A narcotic creates a sedative effect by diminishing the action of the nervous system and vascular system.

Nervine. A nervine calms the nerves or nourishes and tones the nervous system.

Sedative. A sedative promotes calm or induces sleep.

Stimulant. A stimulant is a substance that increases a certain activity. For example, a uterine stimulant may cause cramping or contractions.

Topical. A topical, or topical application, is any remedy that is applied to the skin or outer body.

Vulnerary. A vulnerary is useful in healing wounds.

Suppliers

Herbs and Herb Plants

Adaptations: 808-328-9044

Frontier Natural Products Co-op: **frontiercoop.com**

Garden Medicinals: **gardenmedicinals.com**

Horizon Herbs: **horizonherbs.com**

Medicinal Herb Plants: **medicinalherbplants.com**

Mountain Rose Herbs: **mountainroseherbs.com**

Nature's Cathedral: **naturescathedral.com**

Pacific Botanicals: **pacificbotanicals.com**

Richters Herbs: **richters.com**

Chinese Herbs

Spring Wind Herbs: **springwind.com**

Starwest Botanicals: **starwest-botanicals.com**

Herb Seeds

Abundant Life Seeds: **abundantlifeseeds.com**

Bountiful Gardens: **bountifulgardens.org**

Fedco Seeds: **fedcoseeds.com**

Harris Seeds: **harrisseeds.com**

High Mowing Organic Seeds: **highmowingseeds.com**

Johnny's Selected Seeds: **johnnyseeds.com**

Seeds from Italy: **growitalian.com**

Seeds of Change: **seedsofchange.com**

Seed Savers Exchange: **seedsavers.org**

Territorial Seed Company: **territorialseed.com**

Bottles and Containers

Acme Vial and Glass Company: acmevial.com

Basco: bascousa.com

Berlin Packaging: berlinpackaging.com

General Bottle Supply: bottlesetc.com

Industrial Container and Supply Company: industrialcontainer.com

SKS Bottle and Packaging: sks-bottle.com

Other Supplies and Ingredients

Body Care and Soap Supplies

Botanical Earth: botanicalearth.com

Bramble Berry Soap Making Supplies: brambleberry.com

Columbus Foods: soaperschoice.com

From Nature with Love: fromnaturewithlove.com

Essential Oils

Dreamseeds Organics: hyenacart.com/dreamseeds

Liberty Natural Products: libertynatural.com

Rainbow Meadow: rainbowmeadow.com

Stony Mountain Botanicals: wildroots.com

Herbal Remedies

Great Cape Herbs: greatcape.com

Maine Coast Herbals: maineherbs.com

Motherlove Herbal Company: motherlove.com

Mountain Rose Herbs: mountainroseherbs.com

San Francisco Herb Co.: sfherb.com

WiseWays Herbals: wiseways.com

Vinegar

Bragg Live Foods: bragg.com

Sonoma Vinegar Works: sonomavinegarworks.com

Associations and Schools

Herb Associations

American Herb Association: ahaherb.com

American Herbalists Guild: americanherbalistsguild.com

Herb Research Foundation: herbs.org

National Association for Holistic Aromatherapy: naha.org

United Plant Savers: unitedplantsavers.org

Herbalism Schools

Heart of Herbs Herbal School: heartofherbs.com
(The author of this book, Demetria Clark, is founder and director.)

East West School of Planetary Herbology: planetherbs.com

Herbal Therapeutics: herbaltherapeutics.net

Sage Mountain: sagemountain.com

Wise Woman Center: susunweed.com

Doula Education and Postpartum Doula Education

Birth Arts International: birtharts.com

Recommended Reading

Breastfeeding

Beautiful Babies: Nutrition for Fertility, Pregnancy, Breastfeeding, and Baby's First Foods by Kristen Michaelis and Joel Salatin

Ina May's Guide to Breastfeeding by Ina May Gaskin

The Nursing Mother's Companion by Kathleen Huggins

The Womanly Art of Breastfeeding by La Leche League International

Herbal Remedies for Children and Infants

Childbirth Without Fear: The Principles and Practice of Natural Childbirth by Grantly Dick-Read and Ina May Gaskin

Herbal Healing for Children by Demetria Clark

Pregnancy, Childbirth, and the Newborn: The Complete Guide by Penny Simkin, April Bolding, Ann Keppler, and Janelle Durham

Your Best Birth: Know All Your Options, Discover the Natural Choices, and Take Back the Birth Experience by Ricki Lake, Abby Epstein, and Jacques Moritz

Making Herbal and Aromatherapy Remedies

475 Herbal and Aromatherapy Recipes by Demetria Clark

Aromatherapy for Practitioners by Ulla-Maija Grace

A Modern Herbal (Volume 1, A–H) by Margaret Grieve

A Modern Herbal (Volume 2, H–Z) by Margaret Grieve

Moosewood Restaurant Kitchen Garden by David Hirsch

Rosemary Gladstar's Herbal Recipes for Vibrant Health: 175 Teas, Tonics, Oils, Salves, Tinctures, and Other Natural Remedies for the Entire Family by Rosemary Gladstar

Pregnancy

Ina May's Guide to Childbirth by Ina May Gaskin

Spiritual Midwifery by Ina May Gaskin

Index

Remedies appear in italics.

A
abortion/abortifacients
  Atlas cedarwood and, 23
  boldo and, 24
  comfrey and, 57
  definition, 17, 49, 171
  essential oils and, 22
  mugwort and, 26
  sassafras and, 73
  thuja and, 27
  wormwood and, 74
absolutes, 3–4
acidophilus capsules, 109
acrid, 171
active labor, 135
afterpains and remedies for, 158–160
air freshener spray, 6
air-drying herbs, 42
ajowan, 23
alfalfa, 50
alkaloids, 171
allantoin, 50
allergies
  antihistamine for, 171
  black haw and, 52
  blessed thistle and, 53
  calendula flowers and, 54
  caraway seeds and, 54
  echinacea root and, 58
  elecampane and, 71
  essential oils and, 6, 11
  fennel and, 59
  German chamomile and, 55
  peach leaves and, 63
  PUPPP and, 124
  Roman chamomile and, 55
  strawberry leaves and, 67

  sweet birch and, 24
almond, bitter, 23
aloe vera, 50
alterative, 171
American ginseng, 71
American pennyroyal, 68
analgesic, 171
anemia and remedies for, 91–93, 160–161
angelica
  about, 50–51
  candy recipe, 45
  for delayed placenta, 139
anise/aniseeds
  about, 51
  avoiding, 22
  for heartburn, 114
annual herbs, 39
antianxiety
  citrus essential oils and, 94
  definition, 171
  Infusion, 95
  medications, 93
  Tea, Easy, 95
antibacterial, 171
antibiotic, 171
antifungal, 171
antihistamine, 171
anti-inflammatory, 171
antimicrobial, 171
antinausea
  definition, 171
  Tea Blends (1, 2 and 3), 104, 121
antiseptic, 171
antispasmodic, 171
antiviral, 171
anxiety and remedies for
  about, 93–94
  Bath Oil, Anxiety-Relief, 95

  Diffuser Blend for Anxiety, 94
  during postpartum depression, 156
  Room Spray for Anxiety (1 and 2), 94
  Tea for an Anxious Mother, 151
  while nursing, 148
aphrodisiac, 171
arborvitae, 69
Arcier, Micheline, 2
arnica
  for back labor, 135
  for carpal tunnel, 99
  safety and, 23, 51
  for sciatica, 127
aromatherapy
  for afterpains, 159
  for anxiety, 93–94
  applications, 4
  author and, v–vi
  Back Liniment, Herbal and, 97
  essentials for, 15
  for headaches, 112
  introduction to, 1–2
  pregnancy and, 2, 89
  remedies, basic methods for making, 77–80
aromatic, 172
astringent, 172
Atlas cedarwood, 23
author
  as aromatherapist/herbalist, v–vi
  as doula/midwife, v
  gardening and, 36
  Valnet, Jean, as inspiration to, 2
autumn crocus, 69

B

back labor and remedies for, 135–136
back pain and remedies for, 161–162
backache and remedies for, 96–97
bacterial vaginosis and remedy for, 98
barberry, 69
bark, harvesting, 40
basil
　about, 23–24, 51
　for delayed placenta, 140
　as herbaceous, 14
　safety and, vi
bath oil(s)
　Anxiety-Relief, 95
　Backache, 97
　with essential oils, 78, 109, 118, 126
Bath Tea, Dry Skin, 102
bay, 24
bay laurel, 24
bed rest, for tears & episiotomies, 165
bergamot, 18
Beth root, 51
biennial herbs, 39
birch, sweet, 24
birth of baby, 138
birth of placenta, 138–139
bitter melon, 51–52, 108
black cohosh, 52
black haw, 52, 159
black pepper, 18, 52
black tea, 52–53
black walnut, 53
blackberry leaves, 53
blackstrap molasses, 93
bladderwrack, 69
bleeding, postpartum, 146
Blended Oil for Heartburn, 114–115
blending essential oils, 12–14
blend(s)
　Anemia Tincture, for the Postpartum Period, 161
　Antinausea Teas (1, 2 and 3), 104, 121
　balancing, 13–14
　Canada Fleabane and Cinnamon Tincture, 141
　Epi-Sitz, 166

Extract, for Hemorrhage, 142–143
Lady's Mantle, 140
Pain-Relieving Oil, 128
Tea, for Depression and Fatigue, 156
Tincture, for Afterpains, 160
Transition Tincture, 137
blessed thistle, 53
blocked duct, 153–154
blood clots, postpartum, 146
bloodroot, 69
bloody show, during labor, 134, 135
blue cohosh, 53
blue tansy, 22
body sprays, 4, 78
boldo, 24
borage, 54
bowel movements, during labor, 134
breast care, during breast-feeding, 152–155
breast milk, for massaging cracked nipples, 153
breastfeeding & milk production and aids for, 145, 148–155
broom, 69
broom, Spanish, 24
Broth, Super Nutrition, 105
buchu leaves, 69
buckthorn, 69
bugleweed, 70
bulging tissue, rectocele and, 164
burdock root, 54
butterbur, 70

C

calamus, 24
calcium, preeclampsia and, 123
calendula
　about, 54
　for mastitis, 154
　PUPPP and, 124
camphor, brown, 24
Canada Fleabane and Cinnamon Tincture Blend, 141
Canada fleabane or Canadian horseweed, 54

Candida albicans, 130
candle diffuser, 7
candy, 45
cannabis, 103
caraway seeds, 54
cardamom, 54
carpal tunnel syndrome and remedies for, 98–100, 163
carrier oils
　as diluter, 4
　safety and, 11, 14
　stocking up on, 15
cascara sagrada, 70
catnip, 55, 159
cayenne ointment, 99
cedarwood, Virginia, 25
celery seeds, 75
Chai, Headache, 113
chamomile
　PUPPP and, 124
　Roman, 18
　Tea, 160
chaparral, 55, 70
chickweed, 56, 124
childbirth, 133
chiles, 75
chills, during labor, 137
Chinese, herbals and, 31, 46
Chinese medicine, preeclampsia and, 123
cinnamon
　about, 56
　for gestational diabetes, 108
　Tincture Blend, Canada Fleabane and, 141
citrusy oils, 13
clary sage, 25
cleavers, 56
clove, 22, 56
cocoa butter, for stretch marks, 128
cold remedy, 6
cold-pressing (of essential oils), 3
coltsfoot, 70
comfrey, 56–57, 165
compress(es)
　about, 4–5
　for afterpains, 159
　for blocked duct, 154
　calendula, for mastitis, 154
　for cracked nipples, 153

decoctions for, 81
for hemorrhoids, 115
herbs and, 34, 85–86
for PUPPP, 125
for round ligament pain, 126
for varicose veins, 129
Yeast Wash, 131
Connective Tissue Tea, 163
constipation and remedies for, 100–101, 164
contractions
during active labor, 135
afterpains, 158
during birth, 138
during birth of placenta, 139
during early labor, 134
during transition, 137
coriander, 57
corn silk, 57
cotton root, 70
cottonwood bark, 57, 159
couch grass, 57
cowslip, 70
cracked nipples, 152–153
cramp bark, 57–58, 159
creams (and lotions)
about, 5
arnica, 99
with essential oils, 80
cypress, 18, 22
cystocele, 163–164

D
Dalmatian sage, 23
dandelion/dandelion leaves
about, 58
for constipation, 100
iron in, 91
preeclampsia and, 123
PUPPP and, 124
davana, 22
decoctions, 33, 81
deertongue, 25
dehydrating herbs, 42
delayed placenta and remedies for, 139–141
demulcent, 172
Depression and Fatigue, Tea Blend for, 156
devil's claw, 58
diabetes and remedies for, 107–108

diffuser(s)
Blend for Anxiety, 94
essential oils and, 6–8, 79–80
dill/dill seeds, 58, 114
diluting essential oils, 4
distillation (of essential oils), 3
diuretic, 172
dizziness (and/or fainting) and remedies for, 6, 105–106
dong quai, 51, 70
dosages of essential oils, 11
dried lavender, 118
dropper bottles/droppers, 15
dry skin and remedies for, 101–102
drying herbs, 41–42
Dusting Powders (1 and 2), 168–169

E
early labor, 134
earthy oils, 14
Easy Antianxiety Tea, 95
Ebers Papyrus, 31
echinacea, 58, 109
elecampane, 71
Electrolyte Formula, 104
elemi, 25
emmenagogue, 172
emollient, 172
emotions, during labor, 136
enfleurage, 3
ephedra, 71
episiotomies & tears and remedies for, 164–167, 172
Epi-Sitz Blend, 166
essential oil(s)
as antispetics, for soliders, 2
to avoid, 22–23
Back Liniment, 97
baths with, 78, 109, 118
benefits of, 7
blending/blends, 12–14, 79, 125
breastfeeding & milk production and, 148
buying, 8–10
diffusing, 6–8
expression and, 3
inhaling, 5–6
introduction to, 2–3

pregnancy and, 17, 22–23
for round ligament pain, 126
safety and, vi–vii, 8, 10–12, 14, 17
storing, 12
topical application of, 4–5
types of, 13–14
using, 6
Valnet, Jean, and, 2
eucalyptus, 18
Europe, herbals in, 30, 31, 32
European pennyroyal, 71
Excalibur dehydrator, 42
excessive vomiting and remedies for, 102–105
exotic oils, 14
expectorant, 172
expression (of essential oil), 3
extract(s)
about, 34
angelica root, 139
Blend and Blends 2 & 3 for Hemorrhage, 142–143
with herbs, 82–84
Witch Hazel, 116

F
fainting (and/or dizziness) and remedies for, 6, 105–106
false unicorn root, 71
fatigue and remedies for, 107, 156
feeling/rubbing essential oils, 9–10
fennel/fennel seeds, 25, 58–59, 114
fenugreek, 59, 100, 108
feverfew flowers, 59, 139
flammability of essential oils, 12
flu-like symptoms, during labor, 134
frankincense, 18
freezing herbs, 44–45, 46

G
galactagogue, 172
garlic
about, 25, 59
in the diet, 109
suppositories, 109

Gattefossé, René-Maurice, 2
geranium, 19, 22
German chamomile, 55
gestational diabetes and remedies for, 107–108
ginger, 59, 103
ginkgo, 59–60
ginseng, 71
glass jars, 15
golden ragwort, 72
goldenseal, 72
gotu kola, 60
grades for essential oils, 9
grapefruit, 19
greater celandine, 72
green tea, 99
Group B streptococcus and remedies for, 108–112
gurmar, 60, 108

H
harvesting herbs, 38–41
headache and remedies for, 112–113
healing oils, for stretch marks, 128
heartburn and remedies for, 114–115
heat diffuser, 7–8
hemorrhaging and remedies for, 139, 141–143, 146
hemorrhoids and remedies for, 115–117
herb Robert, 72
herbs/herbals. *See also* specific types of
about, 29–31
for afterpains, 159
for anemia, 91
applications for, 33–35
to avoid, while breast-feeding, 155
for backache, 97
buying, 35–36
for culinary use, 75
equipment for, 46–47
extracts with, 82–83
field guide books for, 37
galactogogues, 149
growing, 36
harvesting, 38–41
herbaceous oils, 14
irradiated, 35
labor & delivery and, 133

organic, 35
preeclampsia and, 123
for pregnancy, 89, 90
preserving, 41–45
quality of, 35
remedies and, 77–80, 81–87
safety and, vi–vii, 32–33, 49
storing, 45–46
teas, 101, 114, 118
timeline, 31–32
vitamin C rich-, 110
wildcrafting and, 36–38
herpes and remedy for, 117
hibiscus flowers, 60
high blood pressure, 123
holy basil, 23
hops, 60
horse chestnut, 60–61
horseradish, 25
horsetail, 61
hot basil leaf infusion, for delayed placenta, 140
humidifiers, 6–7
Hydrating Tea, 120
hydrosols, 4
hypertension and remedies for, 117
hypnotic, 172
hyssop, 25

I
Immune-Boosting Tincture, 112
Increasing Milk Production, Massage Oil for, 152
inducing labor, 134
infused oil/infusion(s)
Antianxiety, 95
for Dry Skin, 102
feverfew flower, 139
for Hemmorrhage, 142
herbs and, 81–82
hot basil leaf, for delayed placenta, 140
to Relax a Breastfeeding Mom, 151
teas and, 33–34
turmeric root, 100
Inhalations for Dizziness, 106
inhaling essential oils, 5–6
insomnia and remedies for, 118–119

internal use, essential oils and, 10
Iron-Rich Tea, Tincture, or Syrup, 91–93
irradiation of herbs, 35
irritation caused by essential oils, 11–12

J
jaborandi, 25
Japanese star anise, 74
jasmine, 25
juniper, 23, 72

K
kanuka, 23
kava kava, 72
kefir, 110
King Henry VIII, 32
Korean ginseng, 71

L
labels for essential oils, 9
labor & delivery, 133
Lady's mantle, 61, 140
lanolin, for cracked nipples, 153
lavandin, 23
lavender
about, 19, 61
essential oil bath, 109, 118
Lawless, Julia, 2
laxative
buckthorn as, 69
cascara sagrada as, 70
definition, 172
rhubarb as, 73
senna as, 100–101
Tea, Herbal, 101
leafy greens, PUPPP and, 124
leaves, harvesting, 40
leg cramps and remedies for, 119–120
lemon, 19
lemon balm, 61, 117
lemon water, 99
lesser galangal, 75
licorice, 61
liferoot (golden ragwort), 72
linden blossom, 23
liniment(s)
about, 5
Back, 162

Back Labor, 136
  decoctions for, 81
  Essential Oil Back, 97
  with essential oils, 80
  herbs and, 34, 84–85
  for sciatica, 127
liquids, stocking up on, 15
lovage, 75
low amniotic fluid and
    remedies for, 120
lozenges, 34, 84, 114

M

ma huang, 71
malta, 149
Mama Milk, 150
mandarin, 19
mandravasarotra, 23
marjoram, 23, 75
marshmallow/marshmallow
    root
  about, 61
  for blocked duct, 154
  for carpal tunnel, 99
  for constipation, 100
  for tears & episiotomies,
    165
  for urinary incontinence,
    168
Mary, Marguerite, 2
massage oil(s)
  about, 5
  for afterpains, 159, 160
  Backache, 96, 162
  Cracked Nipple, 153
  for Increasing Milk Pro-
    duction, 152
  Postpartum (1 and 2),
    157–158
  Round Ligament, 127
  for sciatica, 127
  for Sore Breasts, 152–153
mastitis, 154–155
may chang, 26
medicinal or camphorous
    oils, 14
Medicines Act (1968), 32
melilot, 26
membrane rupture, during
    labor, 134, 135, 137
microwave drying herbs, 43
milk production & breast-
    feeding and aids for,
    145, 148–155

milky oats/oats, 62
minty oils, 14
mistletoe, 72
mixing essential oils, 12
molasses, 93
Mom, Infusion to Relax a
    Breastfeeding, 151
morning sickness and rem-
    edies for, 102–103,
    121–122
Mother, Tea for an Anxious,
    151
Mother's Milk Tea, 150
motherwort, 62
mucilage, 172
mucous membranes, essential
    oils and, 10
mucus discharge, during
    labor, 134
mugwort, 26, 72
mushrooms, 64, 110
mustard, 26
myrrh, 23, 75

N

narcotics, 172
nasturtium blossoms, 109
National Institutes of
    Health, 107
Native Americans, herbals
    and, 31, 32, 37
nausea, during labor, 136
nebulizing diffuser, 8
neroli, 20
nervine(s)
  black cohosh as, 52
  definition, 172
  herpes and, 117
  motherwort as, 62
  PUPPP and, 124
  St. John's wort as, 66
Nesco American Harvest
    dehydrator, 42
nettles
  about, 62
  for carpal tunnel, 99
  for constipation, 100
  for hypertension, 118
  iron in, 91
  for preeclampsia, 123
niaouli, 20
nipples, cracked, 152–153
Nourishing Insomnia Tea,
    119

nutmeg, 26, 75
Nutrition Broth, Super, 105
Nutritional Tea, 106

O

oakmoss, 23
oats/milky oats, 62, 124–125
oil(s)
  Blend, Pain-Relieving, 129
  Leg Cramp, 120
  for mastitis, 155
ointment(s)
  cayenne, for carpal tunnel,
    99
  for hemorrhoids, 115, 117
  plantain, for cracked
    nipples, 153
onion, 26
oregano, 23, 75
organic herbs, 35
oven drying herbs, 43

P

packaging for essential oils,
    10
pain-relieving oils, 128, 155
palo santo, 23
panty liners, for hemor-
    rhoids, 115–116
parsley, 26, 63
passionflower, 63
patch test for essential oils,
    11
patchouli, 20
pau d'arco, 63
peach leaves, 63, 103
pennyroyal, 26
peppermint, 26, 63
perennial herbs, 39
perineum wash, 165
periwinkle, 73
Peru balsam, 23
Peruvian bark, 73
Phytomedicine, 60
pineapple, 99
pipettes, 15
placenta, 138–141
plantain(s)
  about, 63–64
  for cracked nipples, 153
  PUPPP and, 124
  salve, 85, 101
plasters, 34, 86–87
poke root, 73

pollution, wildcrafting and, 37–38
postpartum concerns
  about, 145–146
  bleeding, 146
  blood clots, 146
  depression, 155–158
  hemorrhaging, 146
  remedies for, 146–148, 158–169
  soreness, 146–147
potassium, preeclampsia and, 123
potpourri refresher, 6
poultices, 34, 86
Powder, Yeasty, 131
Practice of Aromatherapy, The (Valnet), 2
preeclampsia and remedies for, 122–123
Pregnancy Teas (1, 2, and 3), 90–91
preserving herbs, 41–45
Price, Shirley, 2
probiotics, 110
prolapses and remedies for, 163–164
protected plants, 38
protein, preeclampsia and, 123
pruritic urticarial papules & plaques of pregnancy (PUPPP) and remedies for, 123–126
pseudoginseng, 71
pulsatilla, 73
PUPPP (pruritic urticarial papules & plaques of pregnancy) and remedies for, 123–126
pushing, during labor, 136

R
raspberry leaves, 64, 91
ravensara, 23
rectal/vaginal pressure, during labor, 137
rectocele, 164
Red Book of Hergest, The, 32
red clover, 64
reishi mushrooms, 64, 110
Relax a Breastfeeding Mom, Infusion to, 151

respiratory problem remedy, 6
rhubarb, 73
rice packs, 135–136, 159
Roman chamomile, 55
Romans, herbals and, 31, 32
rooibos, 65
room spray(s)
  for Anxiety (1 and 2), 94
  with essential oils, 78
  Postpartum, 157
  Transition, 137
roots, harvesting, 40–41
rose, 20
rose geranium, 23
rose hips, 20, 65
rosemary, 20–21, 23
rosewood, 21
round ligament pain and remeies for, 126–127
rue, 26, 73

S
sachet, 118
safety
  essential oils and, vi–vii, 8, 10–12, 14, 17
  herbs/herbals and, vi–vii, 32–33, 49
saffron, 75
sage, 23, 75
salt drying herbs, 43–44
salve(s)
  about, 5
  with essential oils, 80–81
  Hemorrhoid, 116
  herbs and, 34–35, 85
  Simple Stretch Mark, 128–129
  Sleeping, 119
  Varicose Vein, 129
sandalwood, 21
saro, 23
sassafras, 27, 73
sciataca and remedies for, 127–128
sedative, 172
Seed Tea, Milk, 151
seeds, harvesting, 41
senna leaves, 100–101
sex, rectocele and, 164
shaking, during labor, 137
Shanidar Cave (Irag), 31
shelf life of essential oils, 12

shepherd's purse, 65, 140
shittake mushrooms, 110
Siberian ginseng, 71
Simple Stretch Mark Salve, 128–129
sitz bath(s)
  for Bacterial Vaginosis, 98
  with herbs, 87
  Postpartum (1, 2 and 3), 166–167
  for tears & episiotomies, 165–167
  for varicose veins, 129
skullcap, 65–66
sleep, preeclampsia and, 123
Sleeping Salve, 119
slippery elm, 66, 114
smelling essential oils, 9
Smelling Salts, 106
smells and scents, reactions to, 1–2
Sore Breasts, Massage Oil for, 152–153
soreness, postpartum, 146–147
sorrel, 75
southernwood, 73
Soutra Aisle, 32
Spanish sage, 23
spearmint leaves, 66
special needs, essential oils and, 10
spicy oils, 14
squill, 73
St. John's wort/St. John's wort oil
  about, 21, 66
  for carpal tunnel, 99–100
  for round ligament pain, 126–127
  for sciatica, 127
  for varicose veins, 129
star anise, 27, 74
stimulant, 172
stinging nettle, PUPPP and, 124
stocking up, 15
storing essential oils, 12
strawberry leaves, 67
streptococcus, Group B, and remedies for, 108–110
stress and remedies for, 6, 122
stretch marks and remedies for, 128–129

sunlight, as remedy, 153, 165
Super Nutrition Broth, 105
suppositories, 109, 111
sweet orange, 21
syrup(s)
   about, 34
   with herbs, 84
   Iron-Rich, 92
   making, 45

T
Tampon Remedies (1 and 2)
   for Group B Strep,
   110–111
tangerine, 21–22
tansy, 27, 74
tea tree, 22, 109
tears & episiotomies and remedies for, 164–167, 172
tea(s)
   for an Anxious Mother,
   151
   Anemia, for the Post-
   partum Period, 161
   Antianxiety, Easy, 95
   Antinausea Blends (1, 2,
   and 3), 104, 121
   Blend for Depression and
   Fatigue, 156
   Catnip, 159
   Chamomile, 160
   comfrey, for tears &
   episiotomies, 165
   Connective Tissue, 163
   Dry Skin Bath, 102
   Fatigue, 107
   fenugreek seed, 100
   green, 99
   Headache, for Pregnancy,
   113
   Heartburn, 115
   Herbal Laxative, 101
   Hydrating, 120
   and infusions, 33, 81–82
   Iron-Rich, 91
   lemon balm, 117
   marshmallow root, 99, 100
   Milk Seed, 151
   Morning Sicknes, 122
   Mother's Milk, 150
   nettle, 99, 124
   Nourishing Insomnia, 119
   Nutritional, 106
   peach leaf, 103

postpartum, 148, 157
Pregnancy (1, 2, or 3),
   90–91
PUPPP, 126
reishi, 110
Tonic, for Urinary Incon-
   tinence, 169
Yarrow and Shepherd's
   Purse, 140
You Rock! Mama, 147
thrombin, hemorrhaging
   and, 142
thuja, 27
thyme, 27
tincture(s)
   about, 34
   Anemia, for the Post-
   partum Period, 161
   Blend, Transition, 137
   Blend for Afterpains, 160
   Canada Fleabane and
   Cinnamon Tincture
   Blend, 141
   echinacea, 109
   and extracts, 34, 82–84
   Immune-Boosting, 112
   Iron-Rich, 92
Tisserand, Robert, 2
tissue, hemorrhaging and, 141
tone, hemorrhaging and, 141
Tonic Tea for Urinary
   Incontinence, 169
topical, 172
transition (labor) and remedies for, 136–137
trauma, hemorrhaging and,
   141
tray drying herbs, 44
trillium (Beth root), 51
turmeric
   for carpal tunnel, 100
   as safe, for culinary use, 75
   for sciatica, 127

U
ultrasonic diffuser, 8
uncomfortable sex, rectocele
   and, 164
urinary incontinence and
   remedies for, 168–169
US Centers for Disease
   Control, 107
USDA, 38
uva ursi, 74

V
vaginal/rectal pressure,
   during labor, 137
vaginosis, bacterial, 98
valerian, 67
Valnet, Jean *(Practice of*
   Aromatherapy), 2
varicose veins and remedies
   for, 129
vervain, 74
vetiver, 22
violet flowers/violet leaves, 67
vitamin C-rich herbs, 110
vitamin E, for tears &
   episiotomies, 165
vomiting and remedies for,
   102–105, 136
vulnerary, 172

W
Western herbalism, 46
white horehound, 75
white oak bark, 67
wild lettuce, 74
wildcrafting, 36–38
wintergreen, 27
witch hazel
   about, 67–68
   Extract, 116
   for tears & episiotomies,
   165
   wipes, for hemorrhoids,
   116
wood betony, 74
woodsy oils, 14
World Health Organization,
   30
World War I, 32
wormseed, 27
wormwood, 27, 74

Y
yarrow
   about, 27, 68
   for hemorrhoids, 116
   and Shepherd's Purse Tea,
   140
   for varicose veins, 129
yeast infections and remedies
   for, 130–131
yellow dock, 68, 91
ylang-ylang, 22
yogurt, 110
You Rock! Mama Tea, 147

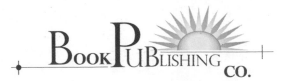
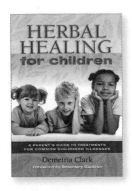
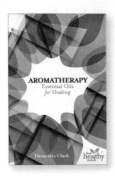
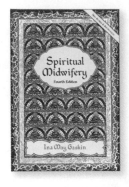
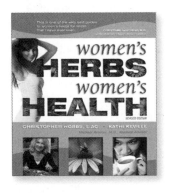
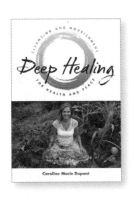
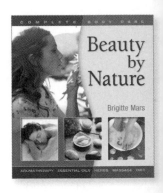